# Solving

# the Enigma

# of AUTISM

# Solving the Enigma of AUTISM

**BY: DR. JEAN-RONEL CORBIER**

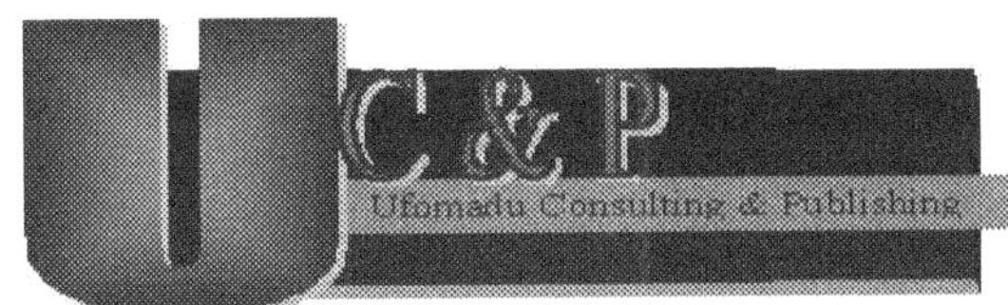

Published by:
**Ufomadu Consulting & Publishing**
P. O. Box 746
Selma, AL 36702-0746

ISBN 0-9754197-2-2
Library of Congress Catalog Card Number: 2004099770

# TABLE OF CONTENTS


ACKNOWLEDGEMENTS 7
PREFACE 9

**PART 1- OVERVIEW OF AUTISM**

CHAPTER 1- HISTORICAL ROOTS OF AUTISM 13
CHAPTER 2- DEFINING AUTISM 19
CHAPTER 3- NEUROLOGICAL CONSIDERATIONS IN AUTISM 35
CHAPTER 4- EVALUATION AND TREATMENT 55

**PART 11- CONTROVERSIES IN THE UNDERSTANDING AND TREATMENT OF AUTISM**

CHAPTER 5- NATURE VERSUS NURTURE 65
CHAPTER 6- THE DAN! APPROACH EXPLAINED 75

**PART III- MAKING SENSE OF AUTISM**

CHAPTER 7- WHY AUTISM IS IMPORTANT 87
CHAPTER 8- ACTUAL CAUSES OF AUTISM 91
CHAPTER 9- MEDICAL PROFILING OF AUTISM 99
CHAPTER 10- OVERCOMING AUTISM VIA THE RESTORATION MODEL 115

SUMMARY 145
APPENDICES 147
GLOSSARY OF IMPORTANT TERMINOLOGY 151
REFERENCES 155
ABOUT THE AUTHOR 161

# ACKNOWLEDGMENTS

I would like to thank God for helping me to complete this book.  I pray that this book will touch many lives.  I would like to give a special thanks to my wife and son for their love, support and prayers.

# PREFACE

A normal healthy infant is born. The parents have high hopes for the infant. The infant does in fact start to develop well, or is advanced. This is a very happy baby. Then, around 18 months of age, something seems to happen. The infant regresses, and no longer is making progress linguistically. The child becomes more and more withdrawn, and starts having annoying tantrums. There are also changes in the feeding habits. The child becomes more particular in his diet. The parents bring their concerns to the pediatrician. Their concerns may initially be downplayed but later, the concerns grow and the parents end up going to see one or two specialists. One day, the scary diagnosis of autism is given. Very little hope accompanies that diagnosis. The frantic research begins and the parents quickly become overwhelmed and confused by the number of treatment options available. They return to the doctor and ask for guidance on the best treatments available. Occasionally, the parents feel that they themselves need some type of treatment because they are at the end of their rope.

Many parents and professionals alike are confused about autism. There are various theories, controversies and approaches when it comes to autism. There are many questions that need to be answered, such as: What is the basic underlying cause or causes of autism? How treatable is autism? Can autism be reversed or cured? Who or what is to blame for autism? Why do many autistic individuals have frequent self-stimulatory behaviors, such as rocking of hand flapping? In what ways are parents of children with autism affected? Which treatments of autism are genuine and which are hoaxes? What can be expected long term for individuals with autism?

With the increase in the diagnosis of autism, it has become an important topic. The increasing prevalence of autism raises several questions such as why are more individuals being diagnosed with autism? Is the increase incidence due to better recognition of the disorder, or are there environmental triggers involved? These questions are important in terms of recognizing the possible contributing and reversible factors in autism.

The purpose of this book is to introduce the reader to the importance of autistic spectrum disorder (ASD). This book provides a comprehensive look at this complex disorder and delves into topics not usually addressed in books on autism. The reader is introduced to a very important model called the **RESTORATION** model. The **RESTORATION** model presents a fresh new look at autism. It also provides a very encouraging treatment approach.

This book will look at autism from a neurological, biomedical, nutritional-metabolic, immune, environmental, genetic, psycho-behavioral and spiritual perspective. This book, in a simple and concise way, attempts to look at autism from all these perspectives. In a broad sense, this book allows us to have a better understanding of the interactions between the intracranial brain, the "gut brain" and the "floating brain" or the immune system. Psychological issues and stressors are all intricately interwoven in the meshwork of autism. Above all, this book provides hope for parents of children with autism. True *restoration* of symptoms for autism and related conditions is believed possible if the right approach is used.

# CHAPTER 1- HISTORICAL ROOTS OF AUTISM

Where did the concept of autism originate?

Autism comes from the Greek word *auto* meaning self. The term *autism* was coined by psychiatrist Eugen Bleuler in 1912. Psychiatrists initially used the term autism to mean *escape from reality*. To say that someone was autistic was similar to saying that someone had escaped from reality, was out of touch with reality, or psychotic. It is this term, *autism* that Leo Kanner used in 1943 to describe a group of 11 children with unique features that describe the disorder we now call autism.

Kanner was in fact the first person to introduce the modern concept of autism. Autism, as described by Kanner, is a condition that has its onset during early childhood. The main characteristic is that of aloofness. Kanner used the term "autistic aloneness". These children described by Kanner appear cut off from their surroundings. In addition, these children have significant language and speech delay and are unable to properly use language as a means of communication. Finally, these children appear to have a persistent need for sameness. They have repetitive movements called self-stimulatory behavior. They are, as it were, prisoners of routine and structure. Though some of these children have mental retardation, Kanner's particular contribution was the delineation of a special group of children with a particular deficit that was unique and separate from mental retardation. What that means is that a child can have autism without necessarily being mentally retarded. Not being able to speak or respond appropriately to social cues is separate from being mentally retarded.

Who was Leo Kanner? He was a psychiatrist originally from Austria. He moved to the United States and eventually went to Johns Hopkins where he practiced pediatric psychiatry. He is credited with having written the first pediatric psychiatry textbook. He also developed the first inpatient pediatric psychiatric ward. Kanner was decidedly a prominent Pediatric Psychiatrist. It is important to realize that autism as described and understood by Kanner was thus primarily a psychiatric condition (Table 1).

## TABLE 1
## Past/Present Labels of ASD

- Infantile autism
- Autistic disorder
- Early infantile autism
- Childhood autism
- Autistic syndrome
- **Triad of social impairments**
- **Autistic psychopathy**

- Pervasive developmental disorders
- **Childhood schizophrenia**
- Asperger's syndrome
- Atypical child syndrome
- **Symbiotic psychosis**

In 1944, one year after Kanner's original description of autism, a German Pediatrician by the name of Hans Asperger described a group of children with symptoms similar to that of Leo Kanner's group. Asperger's group, which was much larger in number, had symptoms very similar to that of Kanner's. Asperger's group was also more diversified. A large subset of children described by Asperger had a *later* onset of symptoms than those of Kanner. Many also seemed to have normal or above normal intelligence. Asperger used the term *autistic psychopathy*. It is interesting to note that both physicians independently used the term autism in their original description, autism and autistic psychopathy respectively. Kanner can, thus, be thought of as the father of autism and Asperger as the second father of autism.

The concept of autism has changed over time. We now have a much broader and more accurate understanding of the nature of autism. Kanner's contribution, however, in delineating autism from the wastebasket category of mental retardation or emotional disturbance is laudable.

In the next few decades autism, which was previously unknown and poorly understood, became associated with some unusual theories. One such theory that was very popular was a psychogenic theory by another prominent individual, an Austrian born American named Bruno Bettelheim. Bettelheim was a developmental psychologist/psychotherapist who had a special interest in childhood developmental disorders. He felt that autism came about because parents, mothers in particular, were cold and distant toward their infants. The psychopathology of the mothers eventually resulted in a cold, aloof, autistic child due to poor maternal-infant bonding. It follows that the proper treatment for such a condition would entail removing these children from that environment and placing them in a more loving, warm and nurturing milieu. This is how the notion of the *refrigerator mother* developed. Mother's of children with autism were described as being cold and unable to form a warm loving bond with their infants. Imagine that after carrying a baby for 9 months and having high expectations for her baby, the mother is then informed that her baby is abnormal and has a dreadful condition called autism. Then, the mother was blamed for it! Bettelheim's theory was actually a prevalent and accepted theory for the cause of autism.

A research psychologist by the name of Bernard Rimland has been instrumental in dismantling Bettelheim's theory, and has supported the notion that autism should be thought of as a biologically treatable condition. Dr. Rimland has in fact started a very important movement called DAN! This stands for Defeat Autism Now! The main objective is to do just that, i.e. Defeat Autism Now! Dr. Rimland, who also started the Autism Society of America, should therefore be called the modern-day father of autism. At this time autism is gaining more recognition, and more individuals are being diagnosed. Many theories have emerged as to why the incidence of the disorder has increased, and the research is ongoing.

18

# CHAPTER 2- DEFINING AUTISM

What exactly is autism? Autism is a condition traditionally characterized by three core abnormalities: that of speech/language/communication, social interaction deficits and behavioral abnormalities. At its worst, children with autism are seemingly cut off from their surroundings. They are unable to effectively interact with their external environment and often have episodes where they appear to be *in their own little world.*

To make matters worse, children with autism often have bizarre behaviors which include self-stimulatory acts or repetitive movements which may include rocking or hand flapping. Autistic symptoms usually start before the age of 3 years.

Autism as a syndrome can be seen in several disorders that seem interrelated. This has led to the psychiatric umbrella term of *Pervasive Developmental Disorders* or (PDD). There are 5 conditions that fall under this rubric:

**PERVASIVE DEVELOPMENTAL DISORDERS (PDD)**

- Autism
- Asperger Syndrome
- Childhood Disintegrative Disorder
- Rett Syndrome

- Pervasive Disorder Not Otherwise Specified (PDD-NOS)

Of these, the only one to occur almost always in females and to have a specific known chromosomal/gene defect is Rett Syndrome. With this condition, an infant who was previously normal, after a few months of age, starts to develop microcephaly (a smaller than normal head circumference). Eventually, the female child develops other cognitive defects and eventually starts appearing autistic. There is a characteristic hand-ringing that develops, representing loss of purposeful use of the hands. Severe seizures usually develop as well as hyperventilation. Dementia sets in early. All symptoms are progressive, making this a neurodegenerative condition. There are several lessons to learn from this particular condition. First, although it is listed in the PDD category, it is a specific condition with a known clinical outcome and pathogenesis. Therefore, any female child labeled with autism who has microcephaly should be worked up for Rett syndrome. Second, most autistic disorders have a male predominance. With Rett's syndrome it is a female disorder. In conditions where there is a male or female preponderance, one must conclude that the sex chromosome are involved. Third, although children with Rett syndrome appear to have characteristics of autism, a specific underlying genetic condition has been identified. Biological/neurological dysfunction, therefore, may result in autistic symptomatology.

Autistic symptoms can be present in a variety of disorders that vary from relatively mild to severe in symptomatology. The term in use now, therefore, is autistic spectrum disorder (ASD). In this book, the term autism and autistic spectrum disorder are used interchangeably. It is important to recognize the early signs of autism so that prompt treatment may be initiated. Below are common examples of early red flags for autism.

**EARLY SIGNS OF AUTISM**

- ## Social Concerns

> Seems to prefer to play alone
> Has poor eye contact
> Is in his/her own world
> Is not interested in other children
> Does not smile socially

- ## Behavioral Concerns

> Tantrums
> Lines things up
> Is oversensitive to certain textures or sounds
> Has unusual attachment to selected toys
> Gets stuck on things over and over

- ## Communication Concerns

> Does not respond to his/her name
> Cannot tell you what s/he wants
> Appears deaf at times
> Does not point or wave bye-bye
> Does not follow directions
> Used to say a few words but now does not

## **CONCERNS THAT WARRANT IMMEDIATE EVALUATION**

No babbling by 12 months
No gesturing (pointing, waving bye-bye, etc.) by 12 months
No single words by 16 months
No 2-word spontaneous phrases by 24 months
ANY loss of ANY language or social skills at ANY age

Let us look at each of the core areas of abnormality in autism more closely. We will start with the one that is most consistently and profoundly abnormal, that is problems with social interaction.

### **Social interaction deficits**

Social interaction deficits are often severe, even in autistic individuals with above normal intelligence. There are two main presentations for social interaction deficits that we encounter in individuals with autism.  In the first category, children are very aloof and are content to be by themselves. This is what led to Leo Kanner's use of the term *autistic aloneness*.  They do not seem interested in other individuals.  They seem quite able to entertain themselves. These individuals, as young children, show little affection even toward close family members. They may spend many hours in their own world. Along with the social aloofness, these children have endless repetitive movements.

Why do the children in the first category prefer to be by themselves?  There are many factors that come into play.  There are impairments that do not allow these children to interact meaningfully with their surroundings. For instance, if this is a child with very severe auditory processing difficulties, including the constant experiencing of painful auditory stimuli, that child will subconsciously learn to shut himself off from the external environment as a coping mechanism. That child will then be forced to turn inward and focus on his internal stimuli. These stimuli may be thoughts, images or other internal signals. As you can imagine, it would be very difficult for a child who is unable to appropriately make sense of the external environment, to socially interact as a normal person. As you might also suspect, the more profound the sensory processing defect, the more significant will be the lack of reciprocal social interactions.

In the second category of social interaction deficit, this subset of children with autism actually seem desirous of interacting with others but obviously still lack the appropriate social skills to do so properly. These children usually are of higher cognitive functioning and will often attempt to be around other individuals. Because they lack very important social cues that make proper reciprocal social interaction possible, their attempts may fail leaving them frustrated, discouraged and sometimes depressed. These individuals may completely lack tact and inadvertently make comments that are offensive. Some even become apologetic after being told what they have said is hurtful. Everything is taken concretely and literally. Humor may be very difficult if not impossible to grasp. Some require constant prompting. These problems make normal social interaction very difficult. These problems may result in a secondary social avoidance because of the severe inability to read and understand social cues. These individuals seem to lack what, to them, might appear as a sixth sense which non-autistic individuals seem to possess.

Children in both categories often have varying degrees of poor or inadequate eye contact. The presence of poor eye contact is very interesting and a look into the cause of this is very revealing. Studies suggest the likelihood that many children with autism who have poor eye contact, are not necessarily trying to *avoid* the face or eyes of the person in front of them. What has been found is that there is a severe impairment in the individual's attention span, such that just as much time may be spent looking at someone's face or eyes as other surrounding objects. On top of that, eye-to-eye gaze may not be used to communicate nonverbally as is the case with individuals who do not have autism.

## **<u>Problems with speech/language/communication</u>**

Children with autism by definition have significant problems with communication. This includes both receptive language (comprehension) and expressive language (speech). Keep in mind that there is a now a spectrum of abnormalities in autism recognizing the presence of lower and higher functioning kids as well as those that fall somewhere in between. This means that some children on the higher end of the spectrum may have relatively mild communication impairment while others, on the lower end, may be severe with complete mutism and apparent lack of any comprehension. Even children with high functioning autism who appear to speak very well with excellent speech may still have subtle language difficulties and deficits. These may include problems with conversational language, that is, there may difficulties responding to questions in an elaborate way. Language may be one-sided and overly focused on the individual's particular set of interests, which may be narrow but profound. There can be deficits in voice inflection and pitch.

Many parents note that language and speech deficits may fluctuate. Even in relatively non-verbal individuals, there may be periods where spontaneous words or phrases emerge, though inconsistent. There may be unpredictable periods of lucidity where comprehension seems better. Along with this variation of speech and language, many autistic children are noted to have unusually strong wills, are stubborn, and like to have things done their way or on their terms. In some emotional states, speech, behavior and cognitive function seem to fluctuate at times to amazing levels. This raises two questions: first, the role of emotional states and cognitive level of functioning in autism and second, the difference between what children with autism will not and cannot do.

## WON'TS AND CAN'TS OF AUTISM WITH RESPECT TO LANGUAGE

How much do children with autism understand? Is it possible that they understand more than we think they do?

- Some children with autism want to speak but cannot.

> It would appear that some children with autism have significant speech impediments that do not allow them to express themselves verbally, although they might have the cognitive ability to do so. There are various mechanisms and biological structures and organs that have to function properly to allow speech to occur. One example would include the tongue. Someone may have the ability to speak but if the cranial nerve or neuronal pathways that control tongue movement are significantly impaired, then speech may not occur. There are similar cases where children with autism can "speak in their mind" but are unable to get the words out. There are other individuals with autism that seem to be able to speak but do so in a very low tone (hypophonic), or they may be able to speak but the articulation may be so poor that what comes out is unintelligible.

Specifically, what are the different speech impediments that interfere with proper communication in children with ASD? In my experience, one often overlooked culprit is the presence of underlying seizures. If a child is having frequent seizures, whether they are obvious, subtle, or even subclinical (i.e. you are unable to see anything externally) that child's seizures may interfere with their ability to speak. Other neurological and cognitive functions may be affected also. Therefore, it is always very important to rule out the presence of seizures in these children. This may entail doing an electroencephalogram (EEG), although in many cases that may not be enough. One may have to do a prolonged sleep-deprived EEG or even a 24-hour video EEG to determine if a child is having seizures.

What are some of the other possibilities that cause speech deficits in a child with autism? An autistic child who is receiving appropriate therapies and where everything is improving significantly (including receptive language skills) but where no progress at all is made with speech, one should always consider, or rule out the presence of a structural central nervous system abnormality. Because of the possibility of seizures or an underlying structural abnormality, it is always important to consider evaluation by a child neurologist. Although a variety of specialists are able to diagnose autism, child neurologists are specially trained to assess and, if necessary, treat *neurological problems* associated with autism such as seizures.

If there is absolutely no evidence of an underlying structural or biological/metabolic abnormality that can account for the child's inability to speak, one has to consider the seemingly strange possibility that the child *can actually speak* but, for a variety reasons **won't** do so.

- Some children with autism do not want to speak but actually can.

  Some children with autism may actually have coexisting selective mutism or may be extremely shy. Selective mutism is a condition where some children who have the ability to speak will do so only in certain circumstances or environments. In my practice, I have been made aware of several instances where a child who is upset or excited enough will actually speak in complete sentences, to everyone's surprise. There are instances were a child with autism will not even attempt to say a word. There are specific reasons for this as well.

Now what would cause a child who has the ability to speak and can do so to remain mute? I believe that most of the children in this category are ones that are exceedingly strong-willed or, as some parents put it, extremely stubborn. These children may be very oppositional and defiant and may express their anger very quickly and intensely. Some of these children may have behavioral or psychogenic impairments that cause their speech to be *suppressed*. There may be some subconscious factors that cause speech to be suppressed the same way that many children with tic disorders are able to suppress their motor tics subconsciously for long periods of time. I suggest that a subset of children with ASD have psychogenic mutism. The underlying processes that account for the behavioral patterns and extreme strong-will may also account for the psychogenic mutism. There are still many things that we do not understand about the human body and especially the mind of young children. It is my belief that even young children can have behavioral and psychological/psychiatric disturbances that can affect various aspects of cognitive and behavioral functioning. Several parents have described what superficially appears to be clinical depression. It may be difficult visualizing a depressed individual who is only 3 years old, but this is possible. The depression maybe caused by endogenous abnormalities. There may be some intrinsic biological defect that is independent of environmental factors. Mood disorders including depression, may be much more prevalent in children with ASD, even in very young, than anyone had expected.

Lack of speech can also be a means of gaining control of one's surroundings. A child can get a lot of attention by not being able to speak, though this attention seeking may be partly subconscious. A child might be able to fulfill various psychosocial needs by suppressing speech that might not be possible if speech were expressed. The underlying factors that would cause such problems in a young child would include a combination of genetic factors, endogenous biological abnormalities, environmental conditions (physical or psychosocial) and the child's particular personality trait. Considering what I stated above, you can see how shyness, selective mutism and autism may involve speech impairments that fall into one continuum. The treatment approach for these children would be different from that applied to children who try very hard to speak but have impairments that are more pathophysiological or structural in nature.

A unique way to view the language problem in some children with ASD is to consider the presence of a severe, biologically based, psychiatric disturbance that causes such a child to be extremely oppositional, defiant, strong-willed, obsessive-compulsive and, on top of that, very moody and quick to anger. In this context, speech, or lack thereof, can be used as a strong agent of manipulation. In some kids, lack of speech represents a form of prolonged ignoring. Of course I am referring to a mixture of psychological and biological disturbances that cause a child to forgo the use of speech. It is possible that if such children were to speak it would not be pleasant ('don't touch me', 'shut up', and 'leave me alone').

There are many children with ASD that are severely affected and truly cannot speak and may not show an outward desire to do so because of the underlying severity of their condition. These children may have varying degrees of cognitive dysfunction/delays.

## **Behavioral problems**

The set of symptoms that cause the most dismay to parents is the behavioral disturbances. This is what leads many parents and doctors to start on the path of pharmaceutical intervention with all types of drugs such as antipsychotics, antidepressants and anxiolytics. The behavior can cause parents to develop stress and anxiety symptoms themselves. This is very important because autistic children often will feed on the parent's distress and anxiety and a vicious interactive cycle begins. Parental anxiety and despair is part of the illness process that complicates autism, although it is hard to avoid.

The cause of behavioral problems must be researched and understood. Therapy and treatment options that simply suppress or cover-up symptoms are not useful and may eventually backfire. Behavior is a function of cognitive deficits, underlying stress and mood disturbances. To understand this, consider what would happen to you if you suddenly became blind for no known reason.

Your behavior would change. You mood would eventually be affected, which would further affect your behavior. In the case of autism, it is a bit more complicated. Imagine a child who does not know that he has an auditory processing deficit. What he hears is significantly distorted. He cannot understand and does not know why he cannot understand. He gets frustrated. It gets worse because outsiders may not know that this child, who may have normal intelligence, is not able to comprehend their words due to a processing defect. This causes the behavior to spiral downward.

Self-stimulation is a specific problem commonly encountered in children with ASD. Sometimes these repetitive behaviors can be so frequent and persistent that they become very annoying. Self-stimulatory behavior can include such things as rocking, flapping, twirling, looking at things from the corner of the eyes, eying things perhaps as an architect would, picking one's eyeball and toe-walking, to name a few. Some self-stimulatory behaviors and movements can be bizarre. These children can have very unusual fascinations and habits such as pica (eating objects like dirt, flowers, leaves or paper). There are various other problems noted. It has been said that individuals with autism have problems getting a lot of things out including:

Emotions- owing to severe social interaction deficits

Words- due to expressive language difficulties

Poop-owing to constipation from gut malfunction

Toxic metals- from an underlying, genetically-based detoxification problem.

Biomedical problems will be more fully addressed in Chapter 6.

## CONDITIONS THAT MAY MIMIC AUTISM

- Selective mutism
- Childhood schizophrenia
- Congenital deafness
- Mental retardation
- Congenital ocular/cerebral visual impairment
- Retrolental fibroplasias
- Septo-optic dysplasia
- Pseudoautism - autistic symptoms caused by lesions in the posterior parietal cortex bilaterally. These children often have an associated disorder of mood and affect. When the mood disorder is treated, communication usually improves markedly.
- Epilepsy-related syndromes
  - Landau-Kleffner Syndrome (LKS)- acquired aphasia (language/speech disturbance) in association with seizure discharges in the temporal/parietal regions.
  - Epilepsy with continuous spike-wave discharges during sleep (CSWDS). This condition is related to LKS.

*It is important to note that conditions that mimic autism may at times coexist with autism making the diagnostic process a challenge.*

# CHAPTER 3- NEUROLOGICAL CONSIDERATIONS IN AUTISM

Is autism a neurological disorder? The answer may seem obvious today, but it is not necessarily straightforward. The most prevalent theory of autism in the past, as mentioned in the first chapter, was psychogenic. How then can we know if this is a neurological condition? We know that autism is a neurological disorder because of the high incidence of seizures in children with autism. **Unprovoked recurrent seizures are always a hallmark of cortical brain dysfunction**. In the general population the incidence of epilepsy is approximately 0.5 %. The incidence of seizures in autism was traditionally found to be at least 30 %. More recent studies that take into consideration the most advanced form of electroencephalogram called MEG (magnetoencephalography), suggests that the incidence is much higher. If you combine children with EEG abnormalities that suggest epileptic seizures with those that have clinical epileptic manifestations the incidence jumps to over 80 percent.

There are two peaks that have been noted for the onset of seizures in autistic children. The first peak is during the toddler years and the second during adolescence. It is very important to realize that seizures can manifest in a variety of ways. Most people when they think that seizures visualize individuals having full body jerking and stiffening with foaming at the mouth and upward rolling of the eyes. This is a type of seizure that many people refer to as *grand mal* seizures and neurologists refer to as generalized tonic-clonic seizures. In reality, there are multiple types of seizures, including several that can be very subtle. Some seizures may present with a brief vacant stare. Some seizures can present with rapid eye fluttering for a brief period of time with no associated alteration in consciousness. Yet other seizures can present with a period of confusion or dazed behavior. Some children have been labeled as being stubborn and are said to frequently "ignore" people. These children may be experiencing brief lapses in consciousness related to seizures. There are laughing seizures, crying seizures, and running in circle or *cursive* seizures. Seizures can also be associated with some disorders that affect speech and auditory comprehension such as Landau-Kleffner syndrome (LKS). Electrographic status epilepticus of slow wave sleep is another condition that can affect speech and other cognitive functions. What this means is that any child who is nonverbal, whether or not there are obvious signs of seizures, should have an EEG to determine whether underlying seizures may be present.

The problem with an EEG, though, is that it is like a snapshot picture in time. Someone who is having seizures but who is having them intermittently may not always have an abnormality seen on routine EEG. This is especially the case with an EEG where no drowsiness or sleep is obtained. For this reason it is always important to obtain a sleep-deprived EEG, especially when seizures are strongly suspected and a previous routine EEG is normal. In some cases one may need a more prolonged study such as a 24 hour ambulatory EEG. The possibility of seizures should always be considered since seizures, when present, can affect behavior, cognitive development and language/speech. In some cases, seizures may directly relate to lack of speech (epileptic aphasia). Seizure medicines are prescribed based on the type of seizure present. Primarily generalized seizures affect the entire brain cortex simultaneously. Partial seizures usually start in one part of the brain and may secondarily generalize.

For generalized seizure disorders:

-Valproic acid
-Topiramate
-Lamotragine
-Zonisamide

For partial seizure disorders:

-Oxcarbazepine

There are several other seizure medications, but these are ones that I have found most useful. It is important that you work closely with a pediatric neurologist when it comes to seizure management and the use of anti-convulsants.

In addition to seizures, we also know that the brain is affected in autism because many children with autism have large heads, or relative macrocephaly. This enlargement of the head is related to brain enlargement. The head size of many children with autism is actually small at birth but then there is accelerated head growth leading to a larger than normal head size in the first few years of life. By adolescence or early adulthood, the head size is no longer larger than normal. This early increase in head size (first few months of life) strongly suggests the presence of an abnormal brain process. Some feel that the increased head size may be the earliest sign suggestive of autism.

What part or parts of the brain are affected in autism? Let us subject the problem of autism to an analysis the way neurologists usually approach neurological disorders. The first question that neurologists always ask is: *Where is the lesion?* In this case, what is the brain localization of autism? The following areas may be implicated based on the clinical manifestations of autism.

*Temporal lobe.*

Children with autism have receptive language problems as well as auditory processing disturbances. Other problems include mood disorders, aggressive behavior, irritability and easy distractibility. All of these problems point to a temporal lobe defect since this lobe is involved in processing of auditory input. It also contains the limbic system which is very important in modulating emotional behavior. The inside part of the temporal lobe (mesial portion) is the most epileptogenic (seizure producing) part of the brain. As we have mentioned, seizures are also common in autism.

*Frontal lobe.*

Many children with autism seem unable to speak, or get the words out. Some autistic individuals who have become verbal report that prior to becoming verbal, they could not figure out how to speak. Lesions or abnormalities in the inferior part of the dominant frontal lobe results in apraxia of speech. The orbitofrontal portion of the frontal lobe can result in impulsive behavior, euphoria, emotional lability, poor judgment or insight, and distractibility. Lesions in other portions of the frontal lobe are responsible for mutism (repetition may be preserved) and outbursts of angry/aggressive behavior.

*Parietal lobe.*

This is often called the sensory cortex. Sensory processing difficulties are common in autism suggesting a parietal lobe dysfunction. A parietal lobe dysfunction can also result in apraxia (inability to perform a command), including a type of apraxia called buccofacial involving impairment in the control of the face and mouth movements.

*Temporoparietal cortex.*

Landau-Kleffner syndrome (LKS) is condition that highly resembles autism but usually has a later onset. EEG abnormalities, pure word agnosias and other clinical findings point to an abnormality in the temporoparietal cortex. Incidentally, there is a subgroup of children with autism that have what neurologists call LKS variant. LKS may actually be on the same continuum as autism. A subset of children with autism may share the same underlying dysfunction as those with LKS, usually an immune/neuroautoimmune disturbance.

*Subcortical structures*

Examples include the basal ganglia, the hypothalamus and other diencephelic structures and the brainstem. These play a role in certain aspects of speech, arousal mechanisms, emotional behavior or affect, repetitive behaviors, regulation of sleep, temperature, the autonomic system and various endocrine functions. Other parts of the brain have also been implicated in autism such as the occipital lobe, the visual cortex and even the cerebellum.

So again the question is: where is the lesion? It appears, based on the above discussion that any lobe can be affected. Consider the problem of attention span, which is a problem seen in most children with autism. Disturbances in attention can be caused by problems in the frontal cortex (prefrontal area), temporoparietal cortex, limbic system and some subortical areas. This means that attention problems likely involve diffuse portions of the brain. When in doubt, we can take advantage of an MRI to look directly inside the brain to see what exactly is going on. The problem is that routine neuroimaging studies are often unremarkable. More detailed studies including volumetric MRIs, functional imaging and even autopsies have revealed some specific abnormalities, but they are inconsistent and varied.

What does all of this mean? Because there is no evidence of a stroke or other visible brain lesion, and because various parts of the brain are implicated clinically, we must strongly consider the existence of a diffuse toxic/metabolic encephalopathy or a global brain dysfunction. This dysfunction may be caused by non structural processes (metabolic, toxic, or nutritional). I believe that instead of permanent brain damage, in many cases we are dealing with a dysfunction that with early, proper, and aggressive treatment may be reversed.

Autism can be viewed as a sort of "Locked-in syndrome". Locked-in syndrome is a neurological condition caused by a devastating stroke or trauma affecting particular parts of the brain. A victim is left without the ability to move, communicate, or respond even though the mind is intact. Such individuals only retain the ability to control closure of the eye. This is their only mode of communication. Similarly, with severe autism a child may be "locked-in". Although the mind may be intact in autism, there are various barriers that *lock these children in*. These barriers are disturbances in sensory, linguistic, behavioral and social functioning. Although speech and language are significant barriers in autism, sensory processing abnormalities can be significant. Sensory disturbances, in particular, hearing distortions or perceptual abnormalities can contribute to many of the limitations seen in autism. Some odd behaviors may actually represent adaptive ways of altering sensory function, whether it is auditory, visual or tactile, to cope with and try to better understand the external environment. Imagine what life would be like if everything other people said sounded like a foreign language. You too would appear socially aloof with altered responsiveness. If you heard explosive sounds, you might have a tendency to cover your ears. The senses are in fact the "avenue to the soul". Visual, auditory, tactile, gustatory and olfactory distortions can affect one's interaction with, and perception of the outside world.

## AUTISM AS A SENSORY PROCESSING DISORDER

<u>Auditory defensiveness</u>

This is one of the most pervasive and often overlooked problems in ASD. Many children with ASD have hyperacute or painful hearing. They can often perceive sounds that normal people cannot. These children, for instance, may hear an approaching airplane long before other people. Unfortunately, various sounds can be very annoying to them and can affect their behavior. In my experience I have noted that many of these children have coexisting central auditory processing disorders. It appears that their auditory acuity is over developed, perhaps at the expense of normal auditory processing and comprehension. There are various auditory based therapies that are aimed at desensitizing their hearing. Hopefully, helping with auditory processing and related auditory dysfunction can improve behavior, socialization and other problems. It is important to keep in mind that, although targeted therapies can often be very useful, this should not completely substitute global treatment interventions since autism is multifaceted.

<u>Tactile defensiveness</u>

Many children with ASD feel uncomfortable when they are touched in certain areas of their bodies. Some children, for this reason do not like to be held and may clearly withdraw from hugs and other displays of affection. One high functioning adolescent boy with ASD explained that receiving a hug, even from a close family member such as his mother, felt like a ton of bricks falling on him. Just as in the case of auditory perceptions, where hearing may be painful, certain tactile stimulation can be very uncomfortable and may in part explain some of the behaviors noted.

<u>Visual processing defects</u>

Vision can be distorted in a variety of neurological and psychiatric conditions including, migraine headaches, Alice-in-wonderland syndrome (where objects have distorted sizes), seizures (where the visual cortex is affected), strokes (where the parieto-occipital cortex is involved), intoxicated states (endogenous or exogenous) and psychosis to mention some examples. The same may apply in some cases of autism. Various objects may appear distorted. In other cases there is some form of light sensitivity. One may have dyslexia or visual agnosia (seeing something without attaching the right meaning, such as a person's face that is viewed as an inanimate object). At least in some cases, these visual perceptual abnormalities may account for the strange manner in which some children with autism look from the corner of their eyes repeatedly. Some children with ASD are apparently able to perceive certain visual phenomena such as a 60 hertz cycle from a light bulb, and fluorescent lighting can be very annoying to them unbeknownst to others. Behavioral optometrists may be able to help with some of these disorders even if a formal eye exam is normal.

## Attention deficit hyperactive disorder (ADHD)

Attention span disorders can be viewed as a form of sensory processing abnormality. Individuals with an attention deficit may not be able to filter out non useful, trivial, or irrelevant stimuli. There is concomitant distractibility. Attention may be so short that it directly affects other areas of behavior such as socialization. For example, the attention given to another person's face or eyes may be so short as to give the appearance of having poor eye contact or eye avoidance. Learning may also be affected. Many children with ASD may come to medical attention, initially, because they are hyperactive and inattentive. Unfortunately, there are many children who are diagnosed late because they come to medical attention specifically for ADHD. While some children have symptoms that respond to stimulants, it is important to be extremely cautious with the use of stimulants in this group. Some children with ASD can have the opposite effect when stimulants are given. Some who also have an underlying tendency or predisposition for tics may have a drastic exacerbation of these symptoms if placed on stimulants. As with other conditions, it is best to identify the patient's nutritional and metabolic status and to make sure that he/she is properly supplemented and is eating a wholesome diet. This should be a priority. In many instances one will find a great improvement with the ADHD symptoms just as with other autistic problems when diet and nutrition are properly adjusted.

## Central auditory processing disorder (CAPD)

A distortion in the comprehension of spoken language can have grave consequences. Imagine that you have perfect hearing but that you cannot make proper sense of what you have heard. In some cases, one may take a very long time to comprehend what is said instead of comprehending immediately. In other cases, one may hear something slightly different from what was actually said, resulting in confusion. We have found that children with auditory processing difficulties often have ADHD and hyperacusis (or painful hearing). In the case of hyperacusis, this can be so unbearable that the young child learns to tune out certain sounds simply as a coping mechanism. Hence, the child appears deaf when not responding to certain sounds, although formal testing reveals normal hearing. CAPD should not be identified with or confused with mental retardation. Many individuals with or without autism may have some degree of CAPD with normal or above normal intelligence. As always, identifying and treating the underlying problem is important and can greatly improve the quality of life for the child.

Sensory abnormalities should always be considered and addressed if found. When properly identified and dealt with, the quality of life may greatly be enhanced. Listed below are a list of therapies and interventions that some parents have reported as useful:

- Auditory Integration Therapy (AIT)
- Tomatis
- Sensory Learning

- ❑ Fast Forward
- ❑ Vision Therapy

Let us look at other neurological abnormalities that can be seen with ASD.

## Headaches

Headaches are likely to occur in a large number of children with ASD, although it may be hard to verify. A lot of children with ASD have somatic and metabolic abnormalities that make them prone to migraine headaches. We know that even very young children can suffer from migraine headaches. Because autistic children are nonverbal or have severely impaired speech, it may be very hard for them to express that they are having headaches. Although not a consistent finding, some very young children with migraine headaches tend to have head banging and sleep disturbances. There are also what are known as migraine equivalents that can be an early indication of full-blown migraines. These migraine equivalents are symptoms that are thought to be related to migraines without the actual presence of a headache. These include recurrent vomiting episodes, bouts of ambulatory instability, and various autonomic and visual disturbances that are transient or intermittent. Some children who have tantrums or spontaneous screaming fits may be experiencing severe headaches. It is very important to consider that proper nutrition is vital not only for the general health of children with ASD, but that nutrition can specifically help with a variety of their symptoms including headaches. For instance, children given caffeinated products to eat or drink may be experiencing exacerbations of migraine headaches due to their diet. Other triggers for headaches may include sleep deprivation, which is often found in children with ASD. Addressing sleep disturbances and ensuring that proper sleep is obtained each night can reduce the occurrence of headaches if present.

<u>Tic disorders</u>

Tics are involuntary stereotypic fluctuating movements or behaviors that tend to wax and wane. Tics can be of the motor type if there are involuntary movements such as frequent eye blinking, or shoulder shrugging. They can also be vocal or phonic if a particular sound is produced. Examples of phonic tics would include grunting, sniffing or other sounds that sometimes can lead to a suspicion of an allergy condition. Both types of tics can be simple (such as eye blinking or a simple vocalization) or they can be complex (more complicated movements such as jumping or saying a phrase with an actual meaning, usually unpleasant ones). Interestingly, some individuals with high functioning autism, because of the presence of significant tics, have been labeled as having Tourette's syndrome when, in reality, they have autism with coexistence of tics. It is important to realize that there is an important subset of children with ASD that have tics. There are also a group of children without ASD that have significant ADHD. Many in fact have all three conditions: autism, tics and ADHD. I believe that ADHD, Tourette's syndrome are part of one spectrum (see Table 2).

# TABLE 2

## AUTISTIC SPECTRUM DISORDER

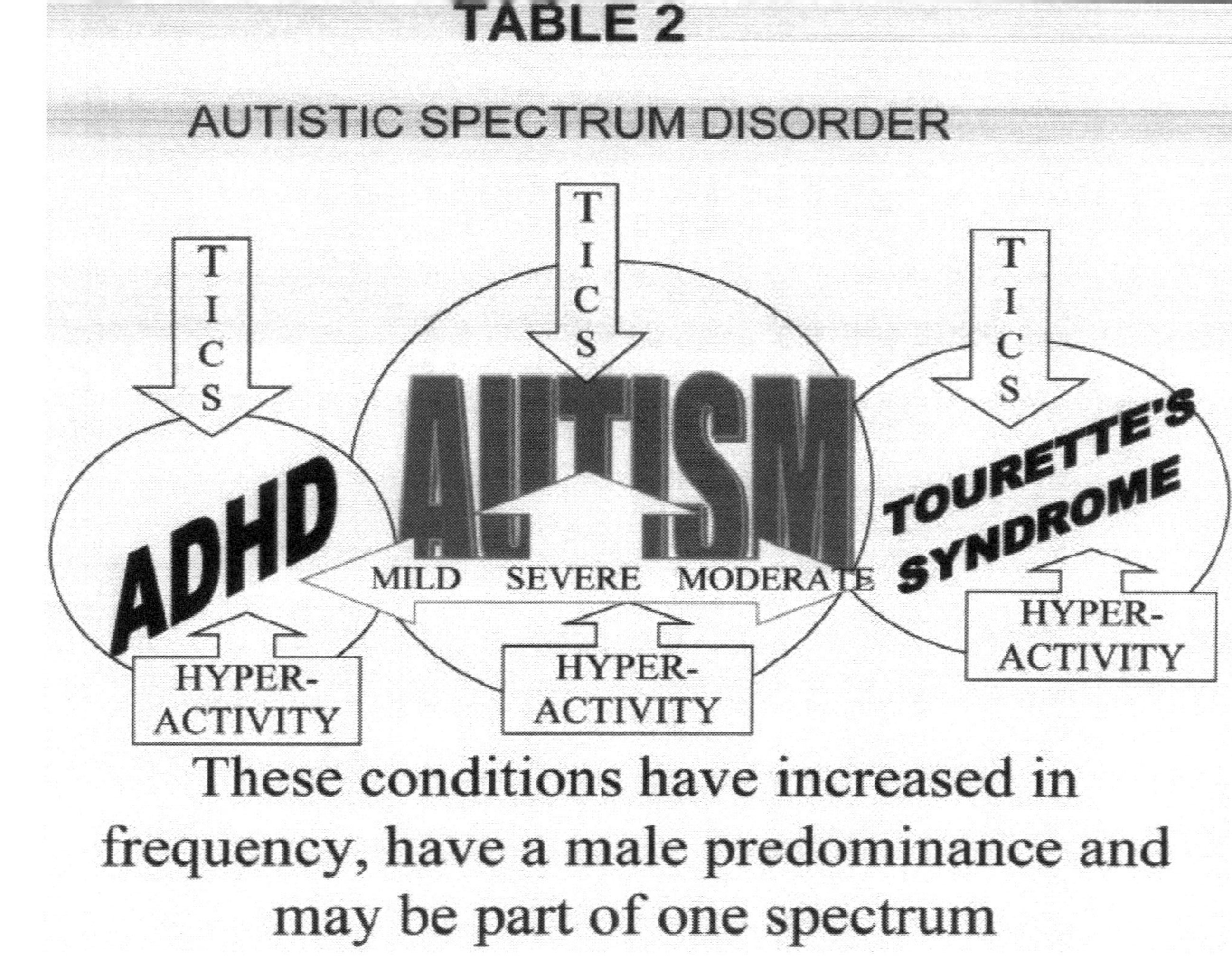


These conditions have increased in frequency, have a male predominance and may be part of one spectrum

## Lack of coordination

Some children with ASD are very clumsy. Many children with high functioning ASD and Asperger's syndrome tend to be very clumsy, although they may have great intellectual and cognitive abilities. There are a variety of reasons why coordination can be impaired ranging from low muscle tone, the presence of very loose/hypermobile joints, or to metabolic/nutritional derangements with subtle structural brain defects. A lot of children may have problems with fine motor skills even if their gross motor skills appear adequate. A good example is handwriting, which can be a problem for many children with ASD. If a child also has coexisting obsessive-compulsive tendencies, which is common, writing can be very difficult. Some children with obsessive-compulsive tendencies are also perfectionists, and tend to rewrite over what they have already written repeatedly. Given that their handwriting is poor or that they may hate writing, this can make any written assignment laborious. I believe that with proper overall treatment of the autistic symptoms, coordination as well as other types of symptoms may improve.

## Sleep disturbance

Many children with ASD do not sleep well. There are a variety of factors that may explain why sleep is impaired. One is nocturnal reflux, pain from headaches or stomachaches, or hormonal/endocrine problems such as low production of melatonin. All of these conditions can interfere with sleep. In some cases anxiety, stress or certain sounds (inaudible to others) can also contribution to sleep disturbances.

Neuropsychiatric disturbances are also commonly present in autism. Keep in mind that they may have an underlying biochemical correlate.

## AUTISM AS AN ANXIETY DISORDER

Most children with ASD have some form of repetitive behavior which, according to the context and manifestation may pertain either to what we call self-stimulatory behavior, tic disorder or compulsion (part of obsessive compulsive behavior). These may fit in the broad category of an anxiety disorder. Certainly, when children with autism are stressed these behaviors may be exacerbated.

Let us look specifically at the problem of self stimulatory behaviors. Self-stimulatory behavior may in part be due to an underlying anxiety disorder, I list below some additional possibilities:

> Self-soothing mechanism/coping mechanism
> Seizure (epileptic or non-epileptic)
> Mode or form of communication
> Movement disorder/hyperkinesias
> Response to internal stimuli

All of the above are distinct etiological possibilities and there may also be a combination of the above factors that accounts for the presence of self-stimulation behavior in children with ASD. These possibilities may coexist and do not have to be mutually exclusive. Motor tics for example, share a lot of features with autistic self- stimulatory behavior. Both may provide a self-soothing purpose. Both can occur intermittently. Both can occur in time of stress or boredom. Both can be exacerbated by infectious illness, and both can drive the parents to distraction.

Most neurologists would not consider self-stimulatory behavior as a manifestation of seizures because motor seizures that originate in the cerebral cortex are usually described as either clonic, tonic or myoclonic. Self-stimulatory movements have a distinct pattern that does not fit into the known seizure patterns. Moreover, an EEG would not likely show an abnormal pattern while these activities occur. One way to view these behaviors, however, is to consider that self-stimulation is a form of **non-epileptic** seizure. Instead of a structural or metabolic derangement causing an irritable cortex, these children may have sub-cortical dysfunctions. These areas that may be susceptible to toxins, neurochemicals, infections, toxic overload from detoxification deficiencies, or hormonal imbalance produced in response to perceived internal stress.

The best way to understand self-stimulation is to understand it in terms of a dysfunction of mental/emotional/psychological origin. This dysfunction affects movement centers in certain portions of the brain resulting in these abnormal repetitive behaviors. Parents and other caregivers must understand that although these behaviors may in part be temporarily suppressed at times they are primarily involuntary movements. It is also important to understand that added stress created by family members or school personnel, can exacerbate the self-stimulatory behaviors as seen in the case of tics. If a child starts having self-stimulatory behavior, the first important step is to identify what possible triggers may exist. Again, these triggers can be toxic-metabolic, nutritional, infectious or emotional. This may happen if the child eats something that does not agree with him, perhaps a food to which he or she is sensitive, or the child may experience a situation that is perceived as very stressful. Things get complicated because what a child with autism may perceive as very stressful, including certain sounds, may be completely irrelevant or even imperceptible to others.

## AUTISM AS A MOOD DISORDER

Mood disorders, such as depression, may be severe in autism. There is even a condition known as pseudo-autism where due to significant depression, a child manifests signs and symptoms of autism. If properly treated, the depression goes away and the child no longer appears autistic. With true autism, however, many children may develop primary or secondary mood changes. In many cases, one may find an extensive family history of mood disorders including in the parents. Mood disorders may be inherited. There are many reasons why a child may eventually develop secondary or reactive depression with autism. Mood changes are important in that they can in part determine behavior and cognitive performance.

## AUTISM AS A PSYCHOGENIC DISORDER

The trauma these children experience can be physical or psychological. A very interesting notion is that some children with autism may have symptoms that are in part related to a psychological or emotional trauma they experienced when they were very young. Children with autism may then be described as having a form of PTSD (Post traumatic stress disorder). In the context of autism, PTSD can also stand for 'post toxic stress disorder' though. Many children with autism become intoxicated by various agents, environmental or dietary. This results in chronic stress and resultant emotional, mood, and anxiety disorders.

Some children with unusual intelligence and memory coupled with a particular emotional genetic makeup are very prone to experiencing long lasting disturbances from an emotional trauma. This trauma may seem trivial to the parents or others but not to the affected child. Psychological trauma can be just as devastating as physical trauma. Both can cause seizures, non-epileptic and epileptic respectively. Both can alter behavior, affect speech and language, cause movement and self-stimulatory abnormalities, and interfere with social interaction. Therefore, both require identification and treatment. We have already discussed the problem of language in this context. Some children with autism may truly have psychogenic mutism where psychological disturbances prevent them from being able to speak. Others may have selective mutism where they speak only with certain individuals and under certain conditions. Of course there are some children with ASD that truly do not know how to speak.

Many children who are neglected or abused may also display autistic features. Fortunately, they may have chronic problems that are completely reversible in the proper environment. This tells us that mind and brain interactions are dynamic and marvelously interconnected. A neglected child can be forced to turn inward as a coping mechanism, and may eventually develop autistic traits. It is known that many institutionalized children demonstrate autistic behaviors, perhaps due to lack of appropriate parental bonding. It is well known that the formative years are very important for future psychological adjustment in life. An interesting idea then is that even young infants, like adults, may be susceptible to psychogenic disturbances that can in part, result in autistic symptomatology.

# CHAPTER-4 EVALUATION AND TREATMENT

Any child suspected of having autism should be evaluated expediently. In some cases an evaluation may reveal that the child has delays that are mild and fall outside of the spectrum of autism. Then there will be situations where the diagnosis will fit the definition of ASD. In any case an evaluation is necessary to make that determination. According to the National Institutes of Health and the U.S. Department of Education, early screenings of children for ASD should be encouraged.

## COMPREHENSIVE EVALUATION OF AUTISM

### FINDING THE RIGHT PEOPLE

#### PHYSICIANS
Primary care physician
Pediatric Neurologist
Child psychiatrist
Developmental pediatrician
Other specialists depending on the case
    Gastroenterologist
    Immunologist
    Endocrinologist
    Geneticist

#### PSYCHOLOGISTS
General psychologist
Neuropsychologist

#### THERAPISTS
Speech/language therapist

Occupational therapist (preferably one trained in sensory integration therapy)
Behavioral therapist/consultant
Physical therapist (for relevant cases)

**EDUCATIONAL SPECIALISTS (Especially those with experience with autism)**

Be aware that autism should ALWAYS be evaluated by medical professionals who can investigate for co-existing medical problems.

**CONDITIONS THAT ARE ASSOCIATED WITH AUTISM**

- Neurocutaneous disorders
    - Tuberous Sclerosis
    - Neurofibromatosis (rarely)
    - Hypomelanosis of Ito
- Congenital endocrine dysfunctions
    - Hypothyroidism
    - Juvenile diabetes
    - Pituitary deficiency
- Congenital hydrocephalus
- Neonatal infections causing encephalitis
    - Rubella
    - Cytomegalovirus
    - Herpes
- Sensory disturbances
    - Deafness
    - Partial blindness
    - Congenital anophthalmos
- Various neurometabolic disorders including:

- o Phenylketonuria (PKU)-
    untreated
  - o Purine/pyrimidine disorders
- Various genetics disorders
  - o Fragile X (most common)

## A DETAILED HISTORY AND PHYSICAL EXAMINATION MUST BE PERFORMED

The history is very important in the evaluation of autism. Parents should be ready to provide the following information to their evaluator:

- Onset of noticeable symptoms
  - o Were abnormalities noted from birth?
  - o Did the child seem normal then regress? When did regression occur?
    - Did any event seem to precede the regression?
- Perinatal abnormalities (e.g. hypoxia, neonatal infection/fever)
- Neurological symptoms
  - o Activity suggestive of seizures (.e.g. staring spells or altered responsiveness)
  - o Coordination difficulties
  - o Progressive cognitive decline
    - This may suggest a degenerative neurometabolic condition
  - o Tone abnormalities
    - Hypotonia (low muscle tone)
    - Spasticity or hypertonia (muscle stiffness)

- o Sensory abnormalities
    - Poor vision (or light sensitivity)
    - Poor hearing (or the opposite, hyperacusis)

- Family history and profile
    - o Family history of ASD
    - o Family history of other neurobehavioral abnormalities (e.g. Tourette's syndrome)
    - o Family history of autoimmune disease (.e.g. lupus, multiple sclerosis, etc.)
    - o Family history of mood disorder (depression or bipolar disorder)
    - o Family history of anxiety disorder (e.g. OCD)
    - o Family history of personality traits (introversion/extroversion/obsession)

It is necessary to have a good general and neurological examination. In addition, the following should be checked:

- Always check the senses (hearing and vision carefully)

    Children with autism may appear deaf, some actually may be.

    Visual changes can result in autistic symptoms.

    Consider seeing a developmental optometrist.

- Always rule out seizures or "epileptic aphasia". A neurologist can perform an EEG.

- Detailed skin examination. Some neurocutaneous disorders are associated with autism such as tuberous sclerosis.
- Check for dysmorphic features which would suggest a possible chromosomal disorder.
- Check tone. Significant hypertonia in the distal lower extremities can point to static encephalopathy (cerebral palsy). These children may walk on their toes.

## 1- NEUROLOGICAL TESTING

- o EEG- this is mandatory since seizures are fairly frequent. Some seizures may be subtle or subclinical.
- o NEUROIMAGING- this is necessary when the neurological examination is abnormal or a structural brain abnormality is suspected. The imaging modality of choice is MRI (magnetic resonance imaging). Imaging may not be necessary in every case.

## 2- METABOLIC TESTING

At the very least the following should be considered:

- o Serum amino acids
- o Urine organic acids
- o Serum lactate and pyruvate
- o Urine uric acid
- o Ammonia

More specialized metabolic tests will be decided by your specialist based on the evaluation such as:

- o Carbohydrate deficient transferin

  One should consider the possibility of a glycosylation disorder (i.e. glycoprotein metabolism abnormality). There are various types of glycosylation disorders. Several are associated with multiple immune dysfunction, gastrointestinal disorders, seizures, speech/language impairment all of which are reported in autism
- o Biotin
- o Acylcarnitine profile
- o Carnitine
- o Very long chain fatty acids
- o Uric acid
- o Purine/pyrimidine disorders Lech-Nyhan Syndrome

There are various other tests that are usually checked by DAN doctors that we will discuss in Chapter 6.

### 3- GENETIC TESTING

- o High resolution chromosomes
- o Fragile X

If there is a significant family history of autistic symptoms and/or dysmorphic features are present you should see a geneticist. In select cases some specific genetic testing (e.g. FISH studies for subtelomeric deletions or other specialized tests) may be warranted.

### 4- GENERAL TESTS

The following may be helpful:

- o CBC (complete blood count)
- o Iron studies
- o Blood glucose
- o Thyroid function tests
- o Chemistry profile
- o Lead level
- o

More specific investigations are necessary depending on specific additional problems that may be present.

## **NON-BIOLOGICAL**

These are gaining more and more acceptance as they should. The ones that are most commonly known and used are listed below.

### **Rehabilitative therapies**

-Speech/language therapy
-Occupational therapy
-Sensory integration therapy -helps correct processing of sensory input to allow effective motor output.
-Auditory integration therapy (AIT) -sound based therapy whereby certain frequencies are filtered out allowing improved auditory perceptual and related functions.
-Sensory Learning - combines multi-models sensory therapies.

### **Behavioral modification therapies**

Applied Behavioral Analysis (ABA/Lovaas) - intensive behavioral therapy that breaks behavior down into *discrete trials*.

### **Educational interventions**

TEACCH -specialized program that helps ASD children maximize the skills they already have.
The Higashi School -a curriculum that focuses on academic skills, fine arts and physical education.

There are various others.

## **Pharmacological interventions**

Antipsychotic agents: e.g. Risperidone
SSRI/antidepressants: e.g. Zoloft
Anticonvulsants: e.g. Lamictal
ADHD medications: stimulants or
Clonidine/Strattera
Other drugs based on symptoms.

Keep in mind that drugs may work but not always. Side effects may also occur. It is always best to search for the underlying cause(s) of the child's symptoms. Indiscriminate, long term use of drugs is not the best approach in dealing with autism. Drugs may play a role in some cases, but they should not be the first option. If a safer and more effective option is available it should be used. When drugs are used, it is best if they are used short term, while completing testing and implementing alternative treatment options which may take longer to be effective.

64

# PART II- CONTROVERSIES IN THE UNDERSTANDING AND TREATMENT OF AUTISM

# CHAPTER 5- NATURE VERSUS NURTURE

Very few medical conditions fuel the type of controversies seen in autism. There are many controversies and polemics with regard to autism. The problem is that these controversies raise serious questions. Well trained physicians and researchers fall on both sides of the fence. The individuals caught in the middle of the controversy are the families of children with autism who are already overwhelmed and are simply looking for safe and effective treatment options for their children. Controversies can serve a useful purpose, however, in that is that they allow us to consider both sides of an issue and to understand subtleties that would otherwise remain hidden.

Some of the main areas of controversy and contention include:

- ❖ The importance of environmental factors versus inherent genetic predisposition
- ❖ The incidence and prevalence of autism
- ❖ Autism as an epidemic
- ❖ The role and safety of vaccines in autism

- o Thimerosal (mercury) and autism
- o The role of the Pertussis vaccine in autism
- o The role of the MMR vaccine in autism
- ❖ The role of nutritional interventions

<u>Here are some recent statistics on autism:</u>

- Prior to 1980 the incidence of autism was believed to be approximately 4-5 per 10,000 for broader autistic spectrum disorder (1/10,000 for classic ASD). The current incidence of autism may be as high as 6/1000 (or 1/150) in some areas.
  - o (CDC, April 2000 "Prevalence of Autism in Brick Township, New Jersey, 1988: Community report"; Report on Autism to the California Legislature)
- There was a 210% increase in the diagnosis of autism in California children over an 11-year period.
  - o (*US. News & World Report,* June 19, 2000, p.47)
- One out of every six children in America suffers from problems such as autism, ADHD, dyslexia and aggression (*US. News & World Report,* June 19, 2000, p.47)

Based on these alarming statistics the following conclusions have been reached:

- ❑ More recent studies found that the rate of autism was higher than the rates from studies conducted in the United States during the 1980s and early 1990s. JAMA 1-Jan-2003; 289(1):49-55 (A study looking at the prevalence of autism in a major US metropolitan area-Atlanta).

❑ Based on reviews of the available literature surveyed, there is evidence of large increases in the prevalence of autism in both the US and the United Kingdom "that cannot be explained by changes in diagnostic criteria or improvements in case ascertainment". Blaxil MF- Public Health Rep-01-NOV-2004; 119 (6): 536-51.

❑ "In recent years concern has been shown about the possible increase in the prevalence of ASD. Studies have shown an increase, but during these last 20 years, diagnostic criteria and definition have also changed. Although many factors are at play, it is evident that there has been an increase". Merrick J- Int J Adoles Med Health – 01 – Jan – 2004; 16 (1):75-8

❑ According to one study, autism is more common in males, multiple births, blacks, increased maternal age and increased maternal education. J Autism and Developmental Disorders 01- June-2002; 32 (3):217-24

Based on the above articles, the reader has the distinct impression that autism is on the rise. Other studies have suggested that there is no major change in the incidence of autism if you correct for certain factors:

> The rates in recent surveys are substantially higher than 30 years ago merely reflecting the adoption of a much broader concept of autism, a recognition of autism among normally intelligent subjects, changes in diagnostic criteria, and an improved identification of persons with autism attributable to better services. Pediatrics Vol. 107 No. 2 February 2001, pp. 411-412.

> "There is evidence that changes in case definition and improved awareness [of autism] explain much of the upward trend of rates in recent decades". Fombonne E- J Autism Dev Disord-01-AUG-2003; 33(4):365-82.

The principle issue of contention in the debate over the increase incidence of autism has to do with possible underlying etiologies. If the incidence of autism is truly increasing at the alarming rate suggested, it means the following:

-Whatever role genetic factors play in the etiology of autism, environmental triggers play an even bigger role.
-If environmental factors play a role, one has to look for environmental changes that have occurred in the past 2 decades since that is when the sharp rise in the incidence of autism has been noted.

- Most obvious changes in the past couple of decades have included:

Increased environmental pollution and toxic exposures.

Increased Thimerosal use (a preservative in some vaccines which contains ethylmercury) as the number of required vaccines for children have increased.

- If the above is true, then clinicians, researchers and politicians must work together to investigate the problem and correct it immediately.

If, on the other hand, the argument that suggests that there is no real increase in the incidence of autism is true, the following applies:

- There is no real need to alarm people about the aforementioned environmental factors in connection with autism.

- Any treatment protocol, based on correcting purported environmental triggers must be erroneous, such as chelation (removing mercury from the body originating from Thimerosal).

- Although more research on autism is needed to determine the cause, the main focus should be on genetics, even if environmental factors play a role.

As we mentioned above, parents are caught in the middle. In a real and practical sense, parents of children with autism want to know if it safe to vaccinate their children, what are the risks, and what should be done if a vaccine (Thimerosal) injury is suspected.  These concerns are valid. Are vaccines safe? Are they contributing to a rise in the incidence of autism?  Some studies have suggested that there is no significant link between autism and Thimerosal. Most pediatricians do not believe that vaccines play any significant role in the etiology of autism.  Some pediatricians are angered because they feel that this sort of controversy can lower compliance rates for vaccination with grave infectious disease consequences to our communities.  Let us look at both sides of the argument concisely and offer recommendations.

<u>Arguments suggesting vaccines/Thimerosal is safe and unrelated to autism:</u>

-Most children who are vaccinated do well and do not develop autism.
-There is no strong proof that the amount of ethylmercury in Thimerosal contained in the vaccines will cause brain injury.
-Genetic studies are revealing increased recognitions of genetic factors:
> e.g. HOXA1 gene and autism
> e.g. 7q22-q33
> e.g. 15q11-q13

The above are a few examples of relatively common cytogenetic abnormalities found (see Appendix C for further examples of chromosomal/genetic abnormalities).

<u>Arguments suggesting vaccines/Thimerosal may be related to autism:</u>

- A study by Dr. Amy Holmes looking at mercury levels in first baby hairs revealed that the levels were actually significantly lower in children with autism, suggesting a mercury detoxification impairment. This in turn was felt to result in higher intracellular accumulation of mercury and therefore organ and brain dysfunction.

- A study entitled "Neurotoxic effects of postnatal Thimerosal are mouse strain dependent" revealed that autoimmune disease sensitive mice subjected to Thimerosal challenges similar to the routine childhood immunization schedule, showed various neurological and neuropathological changes that were not present in other strains of mice without the autoimmune sensitivity. This study suggested that individuals with autoimmune genetic diatheses may be at risk for the development of autism

-It has been noted that a significant subset of individuals with autism have family members with autoimmune disorders.

- The Journal of Pediatrics in November of 2002 published a study entitled "Increased prevalence of familial autoimmunity in probands with PDD". The conclusion in that study was: "Autoimmunity was increased significantly in families with PDD compared with those of healthy and autoimmune control subjects (*those without PDD*). These preliminary findings warrant additional investigation into immune and autoimmune mechanisms in autism".

-In the past, some children exposed to mercury via teething lotions and other mercury containing compounds developed "Pink's disease". This disease had some elements similar to autism, including sensory hypersensitivities and various neurobehavioral problems and acrocyanosis. With removal of mercury, the occurrence of Pink's disease declined significantly.  This suggests that mercury in young infants can lead to autistic-like symptomatology. Some children were noted to be particularly sensitive to the mercury, and others not all.

Given the above information, it seems clear that:

-Autism has a strong genetic component.
-Many children with autism have an autoimmune genetic diathesis.
-Some children with autism may have a particular genetic pre-disposition placing them at risk for Thimerosal/mercury toxicity.

A parent of a child with autism who has a strong family history of autoimmune diseases should be cautious and discuss the above concerns with their physician.

It may be wise to:

- ❑ Postpone all vaccinations if the child is ill.

- ❑ Spread out the vaccine schedule (avoid taking too many vaccines at once).

- ❑ Supplement the child up with multivitamins and antioxidants prior to the vaccinations for extra protection.

- ❑ Use Thimerosal-free vaccines.

- ❑ Any neurological, immunologic or systemic changes noted after the vaccines should be reported right away.

There is nothing wrong with playing it safe until a consensus regarding Thimerosal and its causative role in autism is reached.

# CHAPTER 6- THE DAN! APPROACH EXPLAINED

As a health conscious physician, I have always valued the role of good nutrition in health and the prevention of illness. Based on my background in the field of pediatric neurology, I have also been aware of the connection between the function of the neurologic, gastrointestinal and immunologic systems (see Table 3). I was very happy to learn about a movement called DAN!or Defeat Autism Now, started by Dr. Bernard Rimland. It places a strong emphasis on the role of nutrition, among other things, in autism. I have just discussed the controversies regarding the role of environmental factors in ASD. DAN doctors and researchers, more than any other practitioners, understand the importance of nutritional and environmental factors in autism.

The DAN movement is comprised of a group of doctors and researchers who understand and are devoted to the treatment and eradication of autism. DAN practitioners are good listeners, open-minded, and understand the concerns pertaining to nutrition, vaccination and other environmental factors. Because this movement is so important and many families are trying to implement DAN protocols, and because waiting lists to see DAN practitioners may be long, we would like to explain certain DAN ideas. We always encourage families to seek professional help, but there are certain things that can be done *safely* before you visit a DAN practitioner, if you choose to do so.

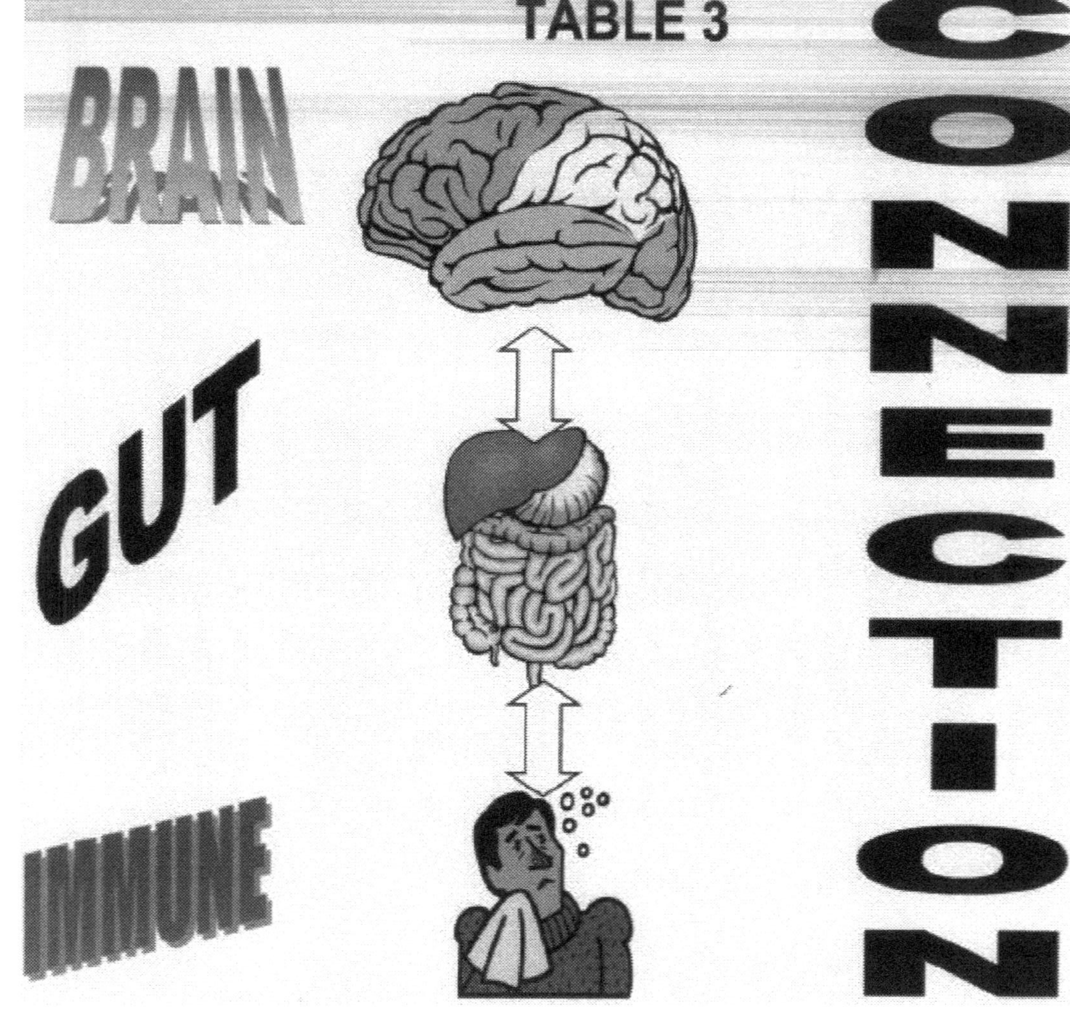

TABLE 3
BRAIN
GUT
IMMUNE
CONNECTION

The DAN philosophy can simply and succinctly be summarized like this:

An infant comes into this world with some genetic vulnerability (immune, metabolic or toxic). After an environmental exposure, such as vaccines/Thimerosal, a susceptible infant becomes injured. This injury may be compounded by the multiple rounds of broad spectrum antibiotics that are prescribed for the child, who seems to have a weakened or disturbed immune system. These antibiotics destroy the balance between good (probiotics) and bad bacteria (pathogens), such that there is an overgrowth of yeast leading to a condition called *gut dysbiosis*. The yeast release various toxins that impair gut activity contributing to a *leaky gut*. Impairment of neurological function due to the release of neurotoxins results. The impaired integrity of the gut wall, allows various macromolecules (improperly digested food substances), toxins and pathogens to pass through the gut wall and into the circulation. This puts a strain on the liver which has to work harder to detoxify these foreign substances. Food allergies or sensitivities develop because the immune system becomes overactive. This further impairs the integrity of the gut wall. As the immune system becomes weaker, the child falls prey to more and more infections with more and more antibiotics given. This leads to a perpetual vicious cycle. Due to oral defensiveness with various textures of food, reflux and other related problems, eating habits become poor, leading to malnourishment. The malnourishment is also due to metabolic disturbances that are innate to the child. Metabolic derangements in various detoxification systems, guarantee an endogenous state of intoxication accounting for many symptoms noted. You then have a child whose immune, nervous and gastrointestinal systems are broken.

Based on the above, treatment of autism entails:

Fixing/healing the gut
Boosting immune function
Nourish the malnourished child while limiting food allergens
Detoxification, this may entail using chelation

<u>A list of the supplements often used:</u>

### -TMG (trimethylglycine)/DMG (dimethylglycine)

> These are very safe substances considered to be food although they resemble B vitamins. TMG is DMG with a third tri-methyl group. Many children with autism have shown improvements with DMG and TMG, a food substance first discovered in Russia. DMG and TMG also have a positive affect on the immune system and possibly on seizures.

### -B6 (high doses) with magnesium

> The effects of B6 and magnesium are well studied. Virtually all of the studies done in the United States and abroad (Europe) have been positive. Several multivitamins designed for

children with ASD have good amounts of B6 and magnesium.

**-Digestive enzymes:**

These allow for the complete breakdown of allergenic food substances (e.g. allergenic proteins that are not completely removed from the diet like casein and gluten). In children with ASD, it is not unusual to see sensitivities to more than 20 food items. Dairy and wheat products are often included in the list for reasons mentioned in the previous section.

**-Colostrum.**

This "nature's food" is a potent natural immune agent that fights yeast and harmful bacteria while providing the right balance of vitamins, minerals, immune and growth factors.

**-Anti-oxidants.**

They inhibit cellular damage caused by the action of free radicals. Many anti-oxidants also protect against heavy metal toxicity.
Coenzyme Q10
Glutathione (oral, intravenous, or transdermal)

Selenium and Vitamin E

Melatonin, this also helps with sleep

## -Lauricidin (monolaurin)

This fatty acid substance is very effective and safe.  It kills yeast/fungi, bacteria and viruses.

## -Cod Liver Oil

Contains both essential fatty acids and vitamin A.

## -Carnosine (CARN-AWARE):

This is a di-peptide of 2 amino acids, histidine and alanine, that are combined. Dr. Michael Chez, a pediatric neurologist from Illinois, has conducted a double blind placebo controlled study with this naturally occurring substance and found it to be very helpful for several of the symptoms of autism, including expressive and receptive language. An open labeled study showed significant seizure reduction in some children that had failed standard anti-epileptic medication. For further information go to www.car-Aware.com .

## -Other amino acid related products

**GABA-** Several anti-epileptic drugs work on GABA receptors in the brain.

**GLUTAMINE-** This helps with immune, gut and brain functions.

**TAURINE AND GLYCINE-** These are abundant in the brain.  Taurine is so abundant and so vital neurologically that it has been labeled a "brain amino acid".

If yeast overgrowth is present, anti-fungal agents can be used

### Natural-nonprescription antifungal agents:

Caprylic Acid
Undecylenic Acid
Citrus Extract
Oil of Oregano
Garlic

### Prescription antifungal medications

Nystatin - safest
Fluconazole
Ketoconazole
Itraconazole
Terbinafine

**Probiotics-** Agents that supply friendly bacteria to the gut to promote its healing.  There are many products available including:

Pro-Bio Gold
Culturelle
Acidophilus
Lactobacillus
Primal Defense

DAN practitioners may do certain tests to aid in the treatment of commonly found biochemical abnormalities.

## **Biomedical testing**

The following tests are useful in guiding biologically based interventions:

**Serum Food Allergy Panel-** This is a blood test that can detect IGG-related food sensitivities that can cause a variety of *delayed* reactions. Depending on the lab used, this test can detect over 100 different food substances that are suspected of causing allergy problems.

**Urine Peptides-** This test provides evidence of partially broken down particles of gluten (a wheat protein) and casein (a dairy/milk protein). This indicates that the individual may not be able tolerate wheat and/or dairy products and that a trial of gluten/casein-free diet is warranted.

**Microbial Organic Acid Test-** There are certain labs that look for evidence of microbial (yeast) byproducts in addition to the conventional organic acids in the urine. This may be the only way in some individuals to suggest the presence of an intestinal yeast problem we call *gut dysbiosis.*

**Comprehensive Digestive Stool Analysis-** This test looks at the various abnormalities that may be found in the gut ranging from yeast overgrowth (and other pathogens) to intestinal permeability dysfunction, so called *Leaky gut syndrome.*

**Heavy metals-** Thee are several ways of measuring the levels of various toxic heavy metals (e.g. mercury, cadmium, etc.) in the body such as hair, blood, or urine samples. The most accurate way of measuring heavy metals in the body is by using a chelator (a special substance that has the ability to bind metal and cause its excretion from the body). Some heavy metals like mercury may leave the blood stream and reside in various tissues in the body, therefore using a chelator is important.

- **Copper, Zinc, Ceruloplasmin and Metallothionein-** These levels and a ratio between copper/zinc can allow the determination of whether a special protein known as metallothionein is deficient. This protein malfunctions in many children with ASD and can be treated to a certain extent with appropriate zinc supplementation.

- o **Essential Fatty acids-** This is a blood test tat is important in ASD children who are picky eaters and those with mood disorders, hyperactivity and short attention span.
- o **Brain autoimmune panel-** There are specialized labs that measure brain auto-antibodies.

**With respect to labs, it is crucial to understand the relationship between an abnormal lab and a clinical manifestation. If, for instance, a yeast problem or casein sensitivity problem is strongly suspected but cannot be substantiated by laboratory findings, the practitioner should still treat the patient accordingly. If there is a positive response to your treatment, your empirical trial becomes the best evidence that there was a problem present. Likewise, an abnormal test does not always translate into a clinical problem. Remember, treat the patient.**

The DAN movement has provided a lot of hope for families looking for answers and safe treatment options. This movement, more than any other, is devoted to the unraveling of the biomedical and environmental factors significant to children with ASD. This movement allies itself with and empowers parents who otherwise feel hopeless, helpless and discouraged. As with every movement, there are some potential problems and dangers. Because most DAN practitioners are very open-minded and willing to work with parents who feel they have a voice, this open environment may foster the introduction of some "unsound doctrines". There are fewer incentives for objective findings. There is a greater danger for 'imposters' to take advantage of families financially. In some cases, erroneous and sometimes dangerous concepts may be passed on by well-meaning but misinformed individuals. Some protocols may become "cookbook" and prescribed for every child with autism, although, in reality the underlying etiologies vary for each child. Finally, sometimes there is such an emphasis on biomedical disturbances, and broader issues are not afforded any attention.

Although I have joined the DAN movement, I have developed a model based on my own understanding of this complex disorder, my experiences and background. This is a model that can be understood and used within other paradigms but also has some unique features. This is discussed in Chapter 10.

# PART III- MAKING SENSE OF AUTISM

# CHAPTER 7- WHY AUTISM IS IMPORTANT

Whether you are a parent of a child with autism, Tourette's syndrome, ADHD, OCD, epilepsy or another neurological/neurobehavioral disorder, it is important to understand the importance of autism (see Table 2). If you are a physician (particularly a neurologist, psychiatrist or developmental pediatrician) or other health professional interested in neurobehavioral disorders, or if you are a therapist, nutritionist or epidemiologist, autism should be of interest to you. Why? Autism is the best example of a disorder that combines neurological, psychogenic, behavioral, emotional, immune, metabolic as well as nutritional disturbances. Some clinicians believe that autism is simply a genetically-based, chronic developmental disorder with its onset in early childhood. Autism is much more than that. Autism is a multifaceted and multifactorial condition. There is reason to believe that in many cases autism is partly iatrogenic, acquired and environmental in origin.

An important interface exists between mind and body and between neurological and psychiatric ailments. Children with autism have both gifts and limitations that redefine our current understanding of the mind and neurological function. Some of the gifts include: *calendar memory* where an individual may be able to name the day of the week that corresponds to any date, years in advance. Some individuals are *human calculators* and can add or multiply and number in their head. Many have perfect pitch. Other gifts and abilities include: photographic memory, artistic talents or amazing musical abilities. Many of these children may have concurrent cognitive deficits that may be severe. Many children with autism are unusually sensitive to things such as foods, weather, criticism, changes in routine, sounds, and fluorescent lights, to list a few. Additionally, they have hypersensitivity syndromes. Many children with autism have poor reactivity to pain, certain auditory stimuli, or environmental stimuli. This suggests that certain portions of the brain are turned on 'high' perception, while other portions are turned down low. This may be a defense mechanism.

Autism also typifies medical conditions that breed controversies. This is the case with disorders that cannot be diagnosed with a laboratory test. Such conditions lead to disputes with respect to their cause, treatment options and etiology. In the case of autism, there is a sharp divide. Some believe in a biomedical paradigm that can explain the cause of autism and whereby biological interventions can be used to treat and sometimes reverse autism. These paradigms look at nutrition and environmental factors, such as vaccines and toxic heavy metals, as playing an important causative role. Conversely, there are others that believe that vaccines, heavy metals, and nutrition have little or nothing to do with autism. Autism, as a genetic and developmental condition, is viewed as a brain disorder which requires pharmacological intervention in palliating symptoms in what is considered a life-long disorder. Reports of "an autism epidemic" and increasing rates are viewed with great skepticism. Alternative explanations are offered such as better diagnosing techniques, revised diagnostic criteria, and greater awareness of the problem. Parents of children with autism are caught in the middle and are often overwhelmed. The problem is compounded by the varied treatment and therapeutic options available. They are purported to be life-saving but may actually be complete hoaxes. How can you tell the difference?

Autism is a disorder with diverse symptoms. In addition to the core diagnostic deficits, many children with autism have seizures, sensory processing disturbances, obsessive compulsive disorder, attention deficit hyperactivity disorder, tic disorders, mood disorders, anxiety disorders, a large variety immune disturbances and gastrointestinal dysfunctions. Despite all of these problems, children with autism usually appear normal physically, and routine imaging of the brain is often unremarkable. This lack of objective laboratory findings has led to some confusion in the classification of this disorder. Is autism a psychiatric, psychological, psychogenic, behavioral or neurological condition? I believe that it is all of the above. Autism is a pervasive condition that causes dysregulation of the highest order in multiple systems of the body. Any approach that fails to take into account the multifaceted nature of this complex condition is inadequate.

# CHAPTER 8- ACTUAL CAUSES OF AUTISM

This chapter is very important because any hope of properly treating children with autism must be predicated on a proper understanding of the causes and contributing factors. Autism, as previously mentioned, is a multifactorial disorder. Its etiology includes genetic, metabolic/nutritional, and post-traumatic factors (the trauma being some exogenous insult). Because the causes of autism are so diverse, it should be viewed at a **syndrome.** This means that various sets of problems that are divergent, can result in the disorder or condition we label as autism.

Any human has the potential to develop autism if the conditions are right. To develop autism you need:

1- A genetic predisposition

Instead of one gene, there are likely a set of genes that must be expressed. If only one or two of these genes are expressed, one may be left with isolated traits such as *toe-walking, auditory defensiveness/sensory processing dysfunction, anxiety/mood dysfunction, shyness* or *sensitive to casein or gluten.* There may be a threshold of genetic dysfunction that must be reached for autism to develop. In some cases, a specific genetic abnormality may be found, but autism is so diverse that it may be futile to chase after "the autism gene". Instead, efforts should be directed toward looking for gene clusters and their interactions in autism.

2- A trigger, trauma or insult

This can range from a viral infection, environmental toxin, or endogenous accumulation of neurotoxins from a metabolic disorder. The trigger may not always be obvious. The 'dose' or intensity of the trigger needed will vary between individuals based on the level of inherited vulnerability. There can be one big insult or several smaller ones combining to create a larger cumulative effect. An insult may also include psychogenic triggers.

3- Proper timing of the insult

The insult must occur early, affecting the developing brain, starting from in-utero up until approximately 3 years of age. Depending on the level of genetic vulnerability, the intensity of trauma and **'other factors'**, one may have mild, moderate or severe autism, with or without mental retardation. One can have severe autism yet be of normal intelligence or can have mild autistic symptoms with co-existing mental retardation. The mental retardation may or may not be related to the autism. What are the **'other factors'** that are important in determining the phenotype of autism? The other factors that are important include:

- Co-existence of a medical disorder
- Overall early health status
- Perinatal complications
- Family support
- Psychosocial and stress factors

- ❑ Nutritional status
- ❑ Lifestyle of family (relative to health)

Autism is a **developmental** disorder specifically because the triggering insult is time-dependent (i.e. it must occur before the age of three). One of the difficulties in autism is that the trigger or insult is not always apparent. The exact timing of the insult is also often unclear.

One factor that deserves our attention with respect to autism is nutrition. The diet of many children with autism is characterized by highly processed foods. There is excessive intake of refined sugar and artificial additive-containing, vitamin/antioxidant/fiber-deprived foods. Most children are addicted to caffeinated beverages and milk, and drink very little water. This sort of diet will eventually cause a decrease in their immunity and defense systems. In June 2002, JAMA reported: "Most people do not consume an optimal amount of all vitamins by diet alone…it appears prudent for all adults to take vitamin supplements." This statement should also include children. They are even more vulnerable than adults because of their brain development and other growth factors that require proper alimentation. In addition to vitamins, various other essential nutrients should be supplemented because they are lacking. Our foods are becoming increasingly processed. There are increasing numbers of artificial food additives that diminish the quality of our food, and ultimately our health. Let us look at just one food substance that is causing a lot of problems and typifies the idea of food toxicology (i.e. toxicological effects from the foods we eat). It is heralded by many as nutritious, wholesome, necessary and natural. Many crave it. I am referring to milk and dairy products.

There are at least 10 reasons why milk is not good for children, especially with autism:

1. It is highly allergenic, causing
   a. Diarrhea
   b. Eczema
   c. Recurrent attacks of nasal congestion
   d. Recurrent bronchitis
2. Many children may not be able to digest milk protein (casein)
3. Some have lactose intolerance
4. It can cause iron-deficiency anemia
5. Associated with so-called "growing pains"
6. Recurrent rashes
7. May cause severe constipation
8. Associated with asthma
9. Associated with nephrosis
10. Milk may be contaminated with hormones and antibiotics.

It is interesting to note that cow's milk is recommended by physician's to be introduced in the diet of children by age one. Children with autism are perhaps more likely than most children to experience the side effects of milk due to their genetic vulnerabilities. Can it be that milk with its problems can trigger a cascade of disturbances that play a significant role in autism? Is there credible evidence that milk and milk products may be harmful?

Many well-known figures including pediatricians and allergists have written about the problems with milk. One such individual is Dr. Frank Oski who wrote the book *"Don't Drink Your Milk"*. Like many, he believes that cow milk is for baby calves and can cause harm in humans. Side effects may range from mild to severe. Dr. Oski has been Professor and Chairman of several pediatric departments including the esteemed Johns Hopkins Children's Center. He has authored hundreds of articles and written several books. He has served on the editorial board of several pediatric journals and was the founding editor of *Contemporary Pediatrics*. A physician and pediatrician of that caliber joins the growing rank of experts that believe that dairy products can cause more harm than good.

A casein allergy, if present, can be a serious problem. Many children with autism have low zinc levels. Zinc is required for the peptidase enzymes that breakdown casein. It is believed and documented by some studies that improperly digested casein will result in peptides called casomorphine. Casomorphine has opiate affects on the brain. This may account, in part, for the increased pain threshold, sensory processing abnormalities, aggressive behavior and "brain fog" commonly encountered in children with autism. There are a lot of alternatives to dairy, including soy, rice and potato-based products for cheese, cream cheese, milk, ice cream, yogurt and other dairy products. Non-dairy products can be found in regular stores. Although nutritional factors are critical to the etiology of autism, there are other non-biological factors that should also be considered in the increased incidence of autism.

Another factor to consider is that we are living in a progressively stressful environment. We have become a very inpatient society. This is the era of faxes and high-speed internet. Everyone is in a hurry. Individualism and materialism is increasing while moral values and spirituality are decreasing. It is possible that these factors may in some part be related to the increased prevalence of autism, mood/anxiety disorders, and other neuropsychiatric conditions. Many children are also not being disciplined properly perhaps due to time constraints, lack of knowledge or other factors.

Someone wrote the following:

Children Learn What They Live

If a child lives with criticism, he learns to condemn.
If he lives with hostility, he learns to fight
If he lives with fear, he learns to be anxious and insecure.
It he lives with pity, he learns to feel sorry for himself.
If he lives with ridicule, he learns to be shy.
If he lives with shame, he learns to feel guilty.
If he lives with encouragement, he learns to be confident in himself and his abilities.
If he lives with tolerance, he learns to be tolerant of others.
If he lives with praise, he learns to be appreciative.
If he lives with acceptance, he learns to love.
If he lives with approval, he learns to like himself.
If he lives with recognition, he learns that it is good to set goals for himself.
If he lives with security, he learns to have faith with himself and in other people.

As we will discuss in the next section, all of these sorts of factors must be considered if proper treatment options are to be implemented.

# CHAPTER 9- MEDICAL PROFILING OF AUTISM

Autism is a very mixed bag. Below are 5 simulated patient presentations of autism that highlight the range of abnormalities that may be present:

<u>Case 1</u>

Raymond is a 35 year old male who lives with his aunt and uncle. He has a job and is semi-independent, but is frequently shadowed by his aunt or uncle because of his problems with social interaction. Raymond is well-mannered and well groomed. He is nice, but socially inept. It is easy for individuals to take advantage of him. He has odd mannerisms and likes to rock back and forth, especially if he is nervous or stressed. He also tends to walk on his toes from time to time but can be walk flat-footed if reminded. He does not like to wear a tie and some times his clothes do not match but he is open to suggestions regarding his dress. He seems to have a photographic memory and can tell you the day of the week for any date that you give him over the next five years. His sense of direction is excellent although at the same time, he does not comprehend some simple things. He can add any number in his head, but cannot solve simple practical problems.

Retrospectively, as in infant, Raymond had mild delays in developmental milestones, especially language. Compared to his older siblings his speech was delayed. This was the first clue that something was wrong. From early childhood, he was found to be very routine-oriented. He thrived in a structured environment, but would have prolonged tantrums if his routine changed even slightly. Some of the tantrums seemed to come out of the blue with prolonged screaming fits. As a child, Raymond liked to line up and stack objects. He had an unusual fascination for certain objects, particularly ones with wheels and spinning objects. Raymond had a tendency to wake up very early, like clockwork. There seemed to be a routine, order and symmetry with everything. The most predictable way to cause a tantrum or meltdown would be to alter these things. His language development was slow, but eventually improved. However, his speech remained laconic and very literal. Eye contact is still poor but improved. Raymond has a cousin who was diagnosed with Asperger's syndrome. For many people who know Raymond superficially, they view him as a nice guy who has some oddities and lack of social cues.

## Case 2

Joanne is now 15 years old. Her main problem at presentation was that of recurrent seizures and speech delay. She also has cognitive delays. The parents' earliest memories are of a very fussy and agitated infant. She was hard to console. All of her developmental milestones were delayed. She initially seemed floppy then became stiff in the lower extremities. As a toddler, she always walked on her toes. Reminding her to walk flat footed did no good, since she was physically unable to do so. She started having staring spells with altered responsiveness at the age of 4 and her first grand mal seizure at the age of 9. She has a least 3 to 4 grand mal seizures per month. She is very clumsy and is in special education classes. She has all of the classical signs of autism and the neurological problems mentioned above. Her neurologist has diagnosed her with cerebral palsy. Her speech is significantly delayed.   There are times when she seems lucid and says some words clearly, that you did not think she knew, but at other times she seems almost mute, usually during her seizures.

In addition to cognitive delays, Joanne has clear evidence of a neurological disorder. She has a cousin with a rare metabolic disorder and a sibling who also speech delays. She has been diagnosed with cerebral palsy but not with autism.   The neurologist has suggested that Joanne may have a neurometabolic disorder presenting with autistic features and cerebral palsy. Further studies have been recommended.

<u>Case 3</u>

David is now an 8 year old male who is well adjusted, mainstreamed in a regular 3<sup>rd</sup> grade and doing well. No one who does not know David's past history, would guess that David had full fledged autism when he was younger. He had been diagnosed independently by 2 professionals when he was age 3, although there were suspicions previously. He started having recurrent ear infections when he was only 4 months of age and was placed on multiple rounds of broad spectrum antibiotics. He was also congested and had very loose stools. He had severe gastroesophageal reflux and was placed on a variety of different formulas as an infant. Despite being sickly, he was doing well socially and linguistically, until between 15 and 18 months of age. There was an insidious but definite change. David became withdrawn and was no longer an affectionate child. He often looked dazed as if in another world. Sometimes he acted as if he were deaf, although subsequent hearing tests were normal. He frequently seemed overwhelmed by certain sounds and crowded situations. He became extremely aggressive, hyperactive and inattentive and overall difficult to deal with. He stopped eating except for French fries and chicken nuggets and seemed to crave cheese and wheat foods. Things started changing when David's parents saw a DAN physician who recommended removing gluten and casein from the diet. The parents decided to undergo a whole lifestyle change. Since both parents and another sibling also have autoimmune disorders and have themselves had recurrent infections, the entire family engaged in complete nutritional changes that have made a remarkable difference in everyone's life.

Although, David initially required speech, occupational, sensory integration and auditory integration therapies, he seems to have overcome his autism. He is now happier, pleasant and turns out to be a very bright, sensitive, affectionate child. Though he has a few problems, his last psychological test shows that he no longer fits within the autistic spectrum.

Case 4

Jeanne and Jane are 15 year old identical twins. Double trouble! Both have been diagnosed with

Asperger's syndrome. The diagnosis was made at the age of 12 years. Previously there were several other diagnoses given by several specialists including: ADHD, OCD, Tourette's syndrome, chronic depression/chronic mood disorder/bipolar disorder, adjustment disorder, oppositional defiant disorder and post-traumatic disorder. The last clinician who made the diagnosis was specialized in the evaluation and treatment of ASD/Asperger's Syndrome and explained why the prior specialists failed to come up with the diagnosis of Asperger's Syndrome.

She explained to the parents that because the girls were very advanced linguistically when they were very young, it would have made such a diagnosis difficult. The parents had also noted that the girls were reading well with good pronunciation by the age of 4. The parents actually were convinced that the girls were geniuses and had high hopes for them. But then, they started to develop signs of hyperactivity, mood changes, and later severe obsessive compulsive behavior. One of the girls, Jane, became so suicidal that she had to be hospitalized in a psychiatric ward for several days. Academically, the girls were straight A students and were found to have very high IQs. They did, however, have significant social interaction difficulties. They lacked tack and got in trouble with their peers because of their comments. When asked how a dress looked by one of her friends, Jane responded that it was the ugliest dress that she had seen. She could not understand why that made her friend upset. She was just telling the truth. Both girls were often melancholic and had severe mood swings that almost became unbearable when they entered puberty. Interestingly, there was a long standing history of mood and anxiety disorder on the maternal side of the family. The girl's father was phlegmatic with little intonation in his voice. He was not very outgoing but, compared to other males in his family he was apparently the most interactive and outgoing.

<u>Case 5</u>

The final individual, Giovanni, is an adult who has never actually been diagnosed with ASD. At one point when he was younger, he was taken to a psychologist because he had significant problems with hyperactivity, attention span and some school difficulties. He did interact socially but was very shy and never initiated a conversation, though he would respond appropriately. He did better with one-on-one interactions than with groups. He did have some autistic symptoms that were mild and apparently spontaneously resolved. Giovanni, who is now a successful chemical engineer, believes that his success can be attributable to a long life of good nutrition, proper family/social/spiritual support and normal brain development. Although Giovanni does not have any family history of autism, there is a family history of ADHD, tic disorder and one individual with chronic illness as a child. That individual had severe asthma, allergies and upper respiratory infections, but was unusually bright with excellent grades in school. There were mild social interaction difficulties and the individual was moody.

The outcome, underlying abnormalities and treatment options vary significantly in each case presented. These cases demonstrate the need for a more effective way to diagnosis ASD. The importance of evaluating autism based on pre-determined categories should maximize the likelihood of proper treatment options for patients based upon the particular category to which they apply. Instead of diagnosing an individual with "autism" or ASD, one might instead diagnose an individual with a specific type of autism representing a specific category applicable to their particular clinical condition.

## PROBLEMS WITH THE CURRENT DIAGNOSTIC SCHEMES

A diagnosis of autism is commonly made based on observation, clinical history and a rating scale, of which there are several. This method of diagnosis relies on identifying a child who meets certain observable criteria based on behavior, communication and social impairments. With such a label, there are automatic images that are evoked in the minds of educators, psychologists, lay individuals and clinicians. These images may lead to certain preconceived ideas regarding proper treatment and prognosis. The problem is that these preconceived ideas may be inadequate depending upon the etiology of autism for a particular individual. It is important, in my opinion, to incorporate information regarding the suspected etiology of autism in developing the diagnosis of autism. Why is this important? If an etiology is considered in making the diagnosis, then treatment protocols can be individualized. Prognostic issues can also be discussed with greater accuracy.

Parameters that should be considered when the formal diagnosis is made include:

> Time of onset of autism. A child who clearly had symptoms from early infancy is different from one who did not show any signs at all until 2 ½ years of age.
> Systemic involvement. For instance, a child who only has communication, behavioral and social deficits is different from a child with accompanying gastrointestinal, immune, or neurological disturbances.
> Presence of regressive symptoms. Some children may have acquired language and social skills normally before 'regressing' into autism. This scenario, as well as the late onset cases, raise the possibility of a toxic, metabolic or iatrogenic cause.

<u>Types of autism:</u>

One way to segregate autism types is based on those that appear to have a primary defect or secondary defect. This latter group can be labeled as having regressive autism, secondary autism or acquired autism.

• Primary or congenital

This group may or may not present with mental retardation. Kanner's original description of autism was likely comprised of individuals in this group. These children may have a congenital defect that may be present even before birth. These are children who may be less likely to acquire speech. There is no obvious regression of symptoms. This group is best labeled as having **primary** or **congenital autism.** They may have some neurometabolic, structural brain defect or specific genetic defect. The goal of investigation in this category is to try to identify a very specific disorder and to treat it as appropriately and as soon as possible to prevent further ongoing damage.

- Secondary or acquired

    Other children with autism seem to have "acquired symptoms" and have been noted to have a regression usually between 1 ½ years of age to 2 ½ years. Many were noted to have normal eye contact, normal social and language develop. Then abruptly, noticeable changes occur. The child starts behaving as if he/she is deaf, looses appropriate eye contact, and may no longer be affectionate. The child may be in a fog state several minutes or hours at a time. Interestingly, in some of these children there are periods of intermittent lucidity. These periods of lucidity may appear haphazardly, during or following an infection, or at other times. These episodes may occur frequently enough to let the parents suspect that there is a potentially normal child that is trapped inside a complex matrix that inhibits proper social interaction, communication and behavior. With these children who were developing normal or in some cases were clearly advanced, one has a sense that there has been an insult to the brain and other bodily organs that have caused the child to change. These children have fluctuations in their symptoms. Some of these children at times may appear normal while at other times, the full characteristics of autism are displayed. The increased cases of autism seen in recent years have in large part reflected children in this category. This group is best labeled as having **acquired** or **secondary autism.** In this group, many individuals may have intact cognitive function and the identification of external factors such as toxins, excessive antibiotic use, specific and food allergy/sensitivities may be more obvious

Another way to categorize autism is to look at predominant biological defects. Based on this model it is possible to come up with a rating system that takes into consideration the various systemic dysfunctions seen in autism. Such a tool would allow a clinician not only to identify potential areas of concern but this would also help decide appropriate treatment. Having a *biological/biochemical autism rating scale* or ***BARS*** would also sensitize families to the areas of dysfunction present.

Examples of categories with an emphasis on biological dysfunction would include (see Table 4):

## TABLE 4

## BIOLOGICAL AUTISM PROFILE

| GUT CHILD | IMMUNE CHILD | NEURO CHILD |
|---|---|---|
| Very colicky as infants<br>Chronic diarrhea<br>Gastro-esophageal reflux<br>Abdominal pain<br>Tantrums<br>Malnourished | Multiple infections<br>-Recurrent Otitis<br>-Recurrent URI<br>-Recurrent Yeast<br>Multiple allergies<br>-Environmental<br>-Food<br>Autoimmune dysf. | Frequent seizures<br>Migraines<br>Focal neurological deficits<br>-Weakness<br>-Unsteady gait<br>Hypotonia or Spasticity |

❖ Gastrointestinal-dominant autism (severe primary gastrointestinal abnormalities)

These autistic children may have chronic loose stools, gastroesophageal reflux, neonatal milk intolerance, fussiness during infancy, leaky gut syndrome, recurrent yeast infections and evidence of chronic malabsorption. These children may do very well with such interventions as the specific carbohydrate and gluten/casein-free diet. Probiotic and antifungal treatment may provide dramatic results.

❖ Immune-dominant autism (severe primary immune abnormalities)

In this group of children with autism there is evidence of immunological problems manifested by recurrent respiratory and ear infections. There may be a strong family history of autoimmune disturbance. Side effects from vaccines/Thimerosal are more likely in this group. Secondary gastrointestinal disturbances may become evident due to overuse of broad spectrum antibiotics and yeast overgrowth. Nutritional interventions, with an aim of boosting immune function, may prove useful (i.e. intravenous glutathione, colostrum, glyconutrients and other strong antioxidants). Intravenous immunoglobulin may especially be helpful for refractory seizures and neuroautoimmune dysfunction.

❖ Neurological-dominant autism (severe neurological problems such refractory seizures)

In this group there may be cognitive delays, frequent seizures, muscle tone abnormalities, severe tic disorders and other evidence of neurological dysfunction. This is the group that should always have an EEG, neuroimaging (MRI), as well as a neurometabolic evaluation looking for specific inborn errors of metabolism. Anti-epileptic therapy may prove very useful. The challenge in this group is to identify the specific underlying problem and treat specifically.

❖ Pseudoautism

There are a variety of conditions that may be permanent or transient that can result in clinical symptoms similar to ASD. These conditions may resolve with time with little need for very specific therapies. There are some children with a diagnosis of ASD that fit in this category whose problem will disappear independent of any treatments or therapies used. Children in this category would include:

Children that have been severely neglected or abused may develop signs and symptoms similar to autism. Although they may have a lot of "catching up" to do, if placed in a caring and loving home, they may normalize. These children may receive speech and other therapies, but the best intervention for them is being placed in a supportive environment. Assuming their brain is healthy, these individuals can normalize.

Other conditions that fit in this category would be children with auditory abnormalities, chronic infections for example. A child with chronic fluid in his ears or chronic infections and associated temporary hearing impairment, has a problem that will interfere with his ability to properly comprehend things. Such a child can appear to have autism. Clearing up the ear infections and having significant improvement in hearing can cause the 'autistic symptoms' to disappear.

Interestingly, there are many children with 'autistic symptoms' that do not meet the criteria for autism or even PDD. Sometimes terms such as autistic "traits" or autistic-like are used. As a parent once asked me, "is there such thing as *borderline* autism?" We have often used the term ***Autistic Equivalent*** to refer to this "borderline" group. An example of this would be the 5th case vignette presented above. These individuals may have autistic symptoms that are not significant enough to cause problems in school or affect self-esteem. Their presentation will not necessarily lead to a diagnosis of autism. These children may fall through the crack diagnostically, but still deserve proper recognition and appropriate support and services.

Parental profiling is also very important when it comes to autism and may provide important diagnostic clues which can be useful for appropriate treatment. Patterns that I have noted in parents of children with autism include:

- Introverted shy/passive/laid back father
- Introverted mother with mild autistic symptoms, sometimes during childhood only
- Primary anxiety and or mood disorder in the mother
- Primary anxiety and or mood disorder in the father

Many parents are noted to be overachievers with an overrepresentation of certain positions and careers, such as CEOs, engineers, architects, doctors, and lawyers. In the case of engineers and architects, one wonders if there may not be some inherited traits that are present in these individuals that have steered them to choose their particular careers, and those traits have been transferred to their children. It is noteworthy that many children with autism have obsessions about symmetry, and behaviors that might suggest a particular neurocircuitry consistent with these traits exhibited by their parents.

In summary, although there are approaches, services and treatment protocols that can be of benefit to all children with autism, medical profiling should be considered since it can help focus treatment options to each individual child.

# CHAPTER 10- OVERCOMING AUTISM VIA THE RESTORATION MODEL

Perhaps the main concern for parents of children with autism is simply finding out what can be done to help their child now! While theories are important and understanding the underlying pathophysiology of the disorder is interesting, parents are concerned with discovering what the best treatment options are for their child. They would prefer to find a systematic, sensible and safe treatment plan that is not financially prohibitive. Dubious authority figures, such as 'Dr. Internet', can be informative, confusing, overwhelming and sometimes misleading. For those families who are 'at the end of their rope', what can be done to help their children recover? Is there reason to hope for a recovery? Is such a thing possible? That is what we want to address in this chapter of the book, which I consider the most important topic.

We have developed a model called the **RESTORATION** model. The term **"RESTORATION"** was chosen since it describes the intent of the model, which is total re-establishment of health and wellness. I use this model not only for autism, but also for other complex neurological and neurobehavioral conditions.

This model is based on the following premises:

- Humans are created beings. God is the Creator and is all

powerful, all loving and all knowing. He is the ultimate healer.

❑ God has created each one of us with self-healing bodies. We are fully equipped with all the tools, processes and the wisdom necessary to heal ourselves when we are sick. These factors also sustain health. We are provided for well.

❑ We are complex beings with a body, mind and soul. We have emotional and spiritual needs as well as more tangible bodily requirements. A disturbance in any of these areas can affect all the other areas.

❑ God has given us a set of natural laws, regulations and guidelines that promote wellness. This is a specific road map or owner's manual to total wellness.

❑ Violation of these natural, God-given health laws place us at great risk for all types of malfunction whether spiritual, physical, behavioral, psychiatric or emotional.

❑ We are designed to be healthy and live long, happy and productive lives. Disease and illness are never haphazard, accidental events, although it may seem that way at times.

- ❑ Total restoration is always possible, although in some cases it would take a miracle. God may in some cases allow illness to occur for the greater good of a patient or family. God is Himself not the author of pain, sickness or anything bad. He may allow this to occur temporarily. Submitting entirely to God's will and His laws is the best way to ensure total restoration. This submission, itself, can be therapeutic. We need to rely upon His will.
- ❑ Because total restoration is possible, one should always maintain an optimistic and hopeful attitude. Patience is often required.

Traditional or conventional approaches are limited when it comes to complex conditions like autism. Focusing primarily on biological disturbances, genetic factors, neurological impairments or other biomedical malfunctions is restrictive. Countless parents of children with autism have been told that the only reliable and proven treatment options are drugs, like risperidone along with proper educational placement. No real hope of cure is provided to the parents. Instead, the parents are told that the child will probably never improve significantly enough to lead an independent life. Some are told to institutionalize their child. This has in fact been a common practice in the past. Many are warned to stay away from any treatment option that includes nutritional interventions because they are not proven to work. Parents are told what approaches to avoid, but not what to do to overcome autism. Autism is not viewed as a curable condition. Officially, autism is viewed as a developmental disorder with an unknown etiology, and no known treatment options beyond simple palliative ones.

The conventional model of medicine as used in general practice today is great in many respects but faulty in others. The medical system in this country is considered by most to be the best in the world, but it is has limitations in certain areas. This is evident in conditions like autism that is commonly viewed as incurable. As mentioned previously, most children with autism have normal brains structurally. Yet, their parents are told that they have a life-long chronic disorder that has no cure. Some cases appear refractory to all treatments. That is because they are viewed from a limited biologically based paradigm, the present conventional bio-medical model. Understanding biomedical factors are vital. In my opinion, these biomedical factors should be understood in the context of normal body physiological function. There is an over-reliance on pharmacological intervention. Ignoring the body's ability to overcome its limitations when it comes to autism, points to some ignorance of the amazing function of the human faculties and their interaction with each other.

In the **RESTORATION** model, we expand the biomedical framework into a biopsychosociospiritual construct. In this construct, biological derangements, which can be congenital or acquired, can alter mental function. But the reverse is *also* true. Acquired or secondary mental disturbances can alter biological function. The immune system is altered by and consequently impacts both biological and mental function. In the latter case, mental disturbances can contribute to impaired immune function also. Social factors are external factors that can also affect health, through their effects on the individual's emotions. Most important, and unique to the **RESTORATION** model, is the central role of *spiritual* factors. The ultimate determination of health and wellness is God's healing power. The spiritual component introduces such concepts as faith, prayer and divine submission. It is because of the spiritual component of this model that makes total restoration possible. Even in cases that are labeled as *incurable, intractable or refractory.* Because this model is based on the premise of a living, all-loving and all-powerful Creator, true hope is encouraged in this model.

Know let us look at the individual components of the **RESTORATION** model more closely.

**The doctor within and the RESTORATION model**

Albert Schweitzer, noted author, physician, missionary and Nobel laureate, once wrote: "It's supposed to be a secret, but I'll tell you anyway. We doctors do nothing; we simply encourage and help the doctor within".

When an ailment is present, one should look for the underlying cause and focus on it for proper treatment. It does not make much sense to treat a condition or symptom, simply by masking it's expression. Here is an example. If someone has headaches that are severe and recur each week, there are two options. One is to take ibuprofen each time the headache occurs. In this first option, one might even take a preventive daily pill for the headaches. By either taking an abortive pill (painkiller) or taking a preventative medication, one is in essence ignoring the actual cause of the headache the drugs are just treating the pain. Ibuprofen makes your headache go away, but this does not mean that your headache was caused by an ibuprofen deficiency. The ibuprofen simply blocked a pain pathway, thereby causing relief to occur. It is important to mention, however, that taking ibuprofen regularly can lead to rebound headaches where the medication itself can cause the headaches.

An alternative approach to treating the recurrent headache disorder is to seek the underlying cause for the headaches and treat it directly. The cause may be nutritional, related to consumption of migraine food triggers such as caffeinated products, processed meats containing nitrates, nutritional deficiencies such as magnesium or riboflavin, or due to a particular food allergy, or to chronic lack of proper water intake. It can be due to poor life style choices such as sleep deprivation or stress provoking factors. Addressing these underlying problems can cause the headaches to go away safely. This does not mean that drugs cannot be used, but this option should be used temporarily and viewed as palliative instead of curative. Identifying the underlying problem and treating it appropriately, however, *can* lead to a cure.

Another example is someone who is always sick with recurrent pharyngitis and upper respiratory infections. One option is to rely on antibiotics repeatedly, which can cause further problems. Conversely, one can focus on boosting the immune system by avoiding foods that are allergenic and overly processed, while increasing the intake of foods rich in vitamins, minerals and antioxidants. The latter is a more natural and safe way to deal with the infections, which may ultimately resolve.

A third example is of a sickly child with multiple allergies and various behavior problems, seizures, headaches and insomnia. One option is to place the child on several drugs. One drug for behavior and a second to counter the specific side effects of the first drug, a third drug to help the child's sleep disturbance, a fourth one for seizures, a fifth drug for the headaches and a sixth drug for treatment of allergy symptoms. A seventh drug is later added to counter the side effects caused by the various drug-drug interactions. This example seems extreme, but polypharmacy (i.e. multiple drug use) for patients is fairly common. A better option is to use *the doctor within* to take care of all of the child's problems which may in fact be interrelated. The child may have headaches and seizures that disturb behavior and sleep, and because of their severity, can cause a secondary mood problem. A better option is using proper nutrition, dietary supplements, avoidance of junk food, and awareness of psychosocial factors that can contribute to sleep disturbances, headaches and mood disturbances.

The popular conventional medical approach of relying on pharmacological intervention as the ultimate solution for everything is unwise. There is virtually a drug for everything. If you are overweight, there is a drug. If you are underweight, there is another drug. If you are sad, there is a drug. If you are mad, another drug exists. If you cannot fall asleep or if you sleep too much, there are drugs for that also. However, there are many drugs that have side effects similar to the conditions that they are treating. Drug therapy can, in some cases, be likened to what we refer to as the *band-aid approach*. When you are bleeding, a band-aid is applied *temporarily* to allow the body to heal itself by causing the blood to clot. Once this occurs, the band-aid can be removed. The band-aid did not cause healing. It only temporarily stopped the bleeding mechanically, while allowing the coagulation cascade to do its job. Drugs, like band aids, may serve a temporary purpose, but, as in the case of blood that clots causing cessation of bleeding, the healing must ultimately come from within.

Children, for instance, who are hyperactive, oppositional and aggressive and are automatically started on stimulant drugs, may not have the actual underlying condition addressed and, therefore, are not being properly treated. Even though some do function better, that does not prove that they had a deficiency of the drug that was given. Even a child that seems to do well on a stimulant drug is at risk for short or long term side effects, and may need several dose adjustments as they continue to grow. Although we are not fond of drugs in general, we do realize that they have a place in patient treatment. The reader must realize however, that many drugs are overused, overestimated in their efficacy, and underestimated in their safety profile. Several "safe" drugs that have been well studied with double-blind, randomized, placebo-controlled, cross over studies are still found later to be dangerous and removed from the market. Many deaths have been attributed to *properly* prescribed drugs. Surely, many people have benefited from drugs, but is that the best and safest approach? Do we over rely on drugs? What about for children with autism? Is drug therapy the answer? It is always rewarding to see a child with autism who has multiple health and behavioral challenges, be weaned off all their prescription drugs and given proper, safe, natural therapies and then do well. There is a place for drugs. When a patient has a seizure disorder I use drug therapy to stop the seizures. For acute or severe recurrent pain syndromes including migraine headaches, we may use drug therapy. Even in those cases, we still think of natural ways of healing.

Pediatric neurologists are aware of seizure syndromes that are very severe and refractory to drug therapy, but respond to natural interventions. A good example is vitamin B6 dependent seizures in infants. This presents with severe, prolonged seizures controlled only by the administration of vitamin B 6 (pyridoxine). Drugs do not work with these seizures. Other conditions include vitamin and mineral deficiencies such as biotin and folinic acid.

Refractory headaches can likewise be caused by specific deficiencies such as that of magnesium. If a child then has idiopathic seizures (i.e. of unknown etiology) that cannot be treated with seizure drugs, can it be that *simple* often overlooked factors may be responsible. With any medical condition, whether neurological or non-neurological, *incurable, refractory, intractable* cases may be ones whose proper treatment approach lies in a completely different paradigm. With biological interventions, it is best to focus on what the body needs, according to my model. Try to identify the underlying problem. If there are multiple problems, concentrate on the primary area of dysfunction, without ignoring the secondary factors and work *with* the bodies natural healing mechanisms. Mobilize *the doctor within*.

Mobilizing *the doctor within* simply means making sure all the natural health laws are followed faithfully. How powerful and competent is *the doctor within* though? To answer this question we have to consider autoimmune disorders. Autoimmune disorders are an important class of medical illnesses. Up to 40 million Americans are thought to have some form of autoimmune disorder including conditions such as rheumatoid arthritis, multiple sclerosis, myasthenia gravis, and Hashimoto's thyroiditis. Interestingly, autism in many cases is now being viewed as a form of autoimmune disorder. Autoimmune disorders are crippling, disabling, and sometimes degenerative in nature. These conditions are examples of the powerful harm that can occur when *the doctor within,* in this case the immune system, attacks the wrong target, which is itself. An immune disorder arises when the immune system starts attacking a person's own organs for example the brain (in multiple sclerosis), the gut (in Crohn's disease), the joints (in rheumatoid arthritis), and the heart, kidneys and brain (in Lupus), etc. The havoc that is brought on by the attack is serious. The immune system is normally there to protect, defend, build up, repair, heal and restore. The proof of its strength is the powerful damage it can cause when its force is unleashed against self.

## Psychosocial factors and the RESTORATION model

Apart from biological interventions, other important factors needed for restoration are, unfortunately, often either neglected or unknown. We live in such a fast paced, high expectation, individualistic society, that it is very easy to get overwhelmed and stressed. There are more and more individuals who develop anxiety and mood disorders. Even young children are having acute 'nervous breakdowns'. In keeping with these problems, I see a portion of children referred to me for neurological problems such as refractory seizures, gait abnormalities, weakness or chronic headaches that turn out to have severe emotional disturbances that account for what appears to be a neurological problem. In other words, seizures do not always have to be neurologic in origin. They can be psychogenic, thereby resulting from an emotional breakdown. Imagine an individual with non-epileptic seizures that cannot be controlled though various drugs are used. It is not that the individual has an incurable case of epilepsy. It is simply that the wrong type of treatment is being applied. This scenario is, unfortunately, all too common. I have encountered extreme cases like a patient whose seizures were so prolonged and unrelenting that the patient was about to be intubated and placed on a breathing machine for the seizures when it was discovered that the seizures were of a psychogenic etiology. The patient revealed to the medical team a life that was very stressful and the patient was at the end of his rope. Stress was converted into an apparent seizure disorder. With appropriate counseling and support, this patient's seizures disappeared completely.

Many children with a variety of behavioral and academic difficulties of unclear etiology may have disorders that are psychogenic in origin. Others may have a very low self-esteem. These children could do well with more support and understanding of their underlying abnormality. Many children get insufficient praise, which they need to thrive. Children need to believe in themselves. Their parents and teachers need to believe in them as well. And children need to know that their parents and teachers believe in them.

I took care of a child who had a lot of problems including severe speech delay. This child was told by other specialists that he would never talk because of the severity of his problems and his age. He was almost 5 years old. I saw him for several visits before he was lost to follow up. I saw him again after a couple of years and was pleasantly amazed to see that he was now speaking well and getting good grades in regular school. I asked the child and parent what made the biggest difference in terms of language improvement. The answer was that he had moved to a new school where everyone believed in him and challenged him. He then blossomed! Interestingly, the child also became healthier. Previously, the child had many illnesses. Yes, I believe psychosocial factors can improve neurological and even immunological function! A happy, secure, relatively stress-free child is much more likely to be healthy than another child who is under a lot of stress with a poor self-esteem, all other factors being equal. Studies in the field of psychoneuroimmunology suggest that mental attitude and emotional status can influence the competence of the immune system, which in turn can alter neurological function. What this means is that a child with autism, who is receiving all of the appropriate therapies (behavioral, educational, and biomedical/nutritional) and that does not make the type of progress expected may have disturbances that are psychosocial in nature holding him back.

The reader should keep in mind that when it comes to biology versus psychology, it is a reciprocal process. Psychosocial factors can have a significant impact on neurological, cognitive and behavioral functioning. The reverse is also true. Biological, nutritional-metabolic or immunologic disturbances can themselves result in emotional and neuropsychiatric disturbances. This is because the brain chemicals that control and regulate our mood and the sense of wellbeing (such as serotonin, the 'happy hormone') require proper nutritional intake for their synthesis. The same can be said of all of the hormones, neurotransmitters or other chemicals that, in some way, are dependent on nutrients such as amino acids, trace elements, vitamins and water for their proper synthesis and metabolism, all of which are indispensable for optimal health.

Hopefully, the reader can begin to see that there are various dimensions and factors to consider when it comes to the treatment of complex neurobehavioral problems such as autism. Restricting and limiting everything to the biological realm is inadequate. Psychosocial factors can be just as important. Psychosocial factors are not just important for the patient but for parents as well since they are ipso facto enmeshed in their child's illness. In a broad sense, it may be said that the child's illness extends to the parents. The child's anxiety may also be the parent's anxiety. The child's stress is also the parent's stress. The learned helplessness and pessimism may also become that of the parents'. This will add an additional component to the child's stress, further compounding their overall stress Proper restoration then may entail the need for positive changes that are experienced not only by the sick child, but also by the affected parents, neighbors and everyone involved with the child.

The final and most important realm to consider pertaining to the RESTORATION model is the spiritual component.

## Spiritual factors and the RESTORATION model

This spiritual portion of the **RESTORATION** model is the most crucial and unique. Many psychosocial disturbances may involve spiritual dysfunction as well. It is interesting that even the Diagnostic and Statistical Manual Mental Disorder fourth edition (DSM-IV) acknowledges the role of religious dysfunction in mental health. With spiritual matters we start delving into the "Why" questions. Why is a particular child born with a severe genetic disorder? Why is your child affected and not another? Why does God allow certain bad things to happen to good people? What about hope, prayer and faith? What role do they play or should they play in medicine, especially when dealing with disorders such as autism?

In Genesis 1: 29 in the Bible, God informed Adam and Eve that their diet should specifically consist of "every seed bearing-plant on the face of all the earth and every tree that has fruit with seed in it." He said furthermore "they will be yours for food". This statement has far-reaching implications for us. First of all it entails believing in a Creator. One must consider that the Creator specifically designed our body to function properly and has provided an operator's manual. In other words, by following a specific divine nutritional prescription, the goal was for the body to function impeccably. So what does all of this have to do with autism? And, how does this pertain to spirituality? God has provided us with special nutrients that He created that would not only feed the body, but would also allow optimal spiritual development so that man could be at his best physically, psychologically and spiritually. God knew that a body that was not well nourished would result in improper functioning of the brain, which is the organ of the mind and, hence the patient's spirituality would ultimately be compromised. Feeding the body properly, therefore, by following God's initial dietary prescription, would result first in biological health and, ultimately in spiritual wellness. Thus, it is important for us to take good care of our bodies. Based on the fact that man was initially given for food "every seed bearing-plant on the face of the earth and every tree that has fruit with seed in it" it is logical to think that God has placed in nature everything the body needs to function properly. When considering autism today and looking at most children's diet, how closely is it to God's original prescription for health? What would happen if these laws *were* applied in the lives of children with autism? What do fruits and herbs and vegetables contain that could restore children with autism?

It is interesting to note that fresh, raw, ripely-picked fruits and vegetables contain an impressive assortment of vitamins, minerals, antioxidants, fiber, water and perhaps thousands of phytochemicals that the nervous system and the rest of the body need to function properly. It should not be a surprise from a nutritional standpoint that if children with ASD ate daily ALL of the required servings of raw fruits and vegetables, that they were harvested from a rich soil, ripely-picked and pesticide-free, with the required amount of water the body needs, these children would function at a much higher level. The sad reality is that most autistic kids are very picky eaters and have various oral sensory and texture limitations to certain foods. Instead of eating the foods needed, these children seem addicted to the common U.S. pediatric diet of junk food. The favorite meat source is chicken nuggets. These foods are given to the children not because they are healthy but because the children demand these foods. Many of these children who are receiving behavioral therapies receive candy or other refined sugars products as a source of reward.

God's natural laws also include *spiritual* foods such as faith, prayer, humility, patience, joy and hope. Faith is the belief that God has the power to heal. God's power starts where our strength ends. Faith, properly understood, has several components including: the *fear of the Lord,* abiding by His precepts, and asking for healing. Christ says "ask and it will be given to you". With faith one has to be persistent. Faith also entails implicit trust in God. It is alright to place your faith in doctors, various interventions and drugs, as long as you understand that all of these have their limitations. Why not place your faith in God, who has the power to heal and restore. He created us, and, if necessary can 'recreate' us. Finally, with faith there is an element of time. Not our time, but God's. What would you do today if your child could suddenly talk? How would you behave if your child were restored to normal? God can make that happen, if He so desires, and if you are ready to give Him the praise, and if that experience will draw you closer to God.

Prayer is an important gateway to God's throne. Prayer and faith are important tools, necessary for restoration to occur. When God is ready to heal, He is not interested in the timing of an injury, whether the damage is permanent or not, what specialists have already been seen, how soon interventions were started, what the mechanism of injury is or what co-existing problems are present. He is only interested in the quality of your faith and the sincerity of your prayer request. Some lack humility, and are arrogant. It is impossible to please God if one lacks faith and humility.

As a physician and specialist, I have never been afraid to call on Christ for help. There have been medical situations where I desperately needed His help and He gave it to me in a miraculous way. One particular case was of a patient who was admitted to the intensive care unit while I was on call. The patient went into an acute coma of undetermined etiology. I was contacted and ordered several tests. We were able to diagnosis a condition called acute disseminated encephalomyelitis where the brain and spine swell. This can be a serious condition, as it was in this case. Because of the brain swelling, the patient developed increased pressure inside the skull to the point where a monitor was inserted through the skull. Unfortunately, the pressure kept rising until it was believed that death was imminent. The patient was in a deep coma, on a breathing machine with a catheter stuck through the skull. There was evidence of frequent seizures on the EEG. The prognosis was poor. One morning when I made my rounds, I felt like I needed to avoid the parents since I had no good news to offer. Our best efforts seemed futile. As I wrote my note on the chart, the parent approached me and desperately cried "if there is anything you can do to help my child, if you need to call on God's name, anything for my child". I must admit that I had not considered prayer up to that point, nor did the parent know about my religious beliefs. I asked "do you have faith in God's ability to heal." The answer was yes. With that, I held the parent's hands, asking God to heal and to restore the child, if it was His will. It was a short and simple prayer. I told the parents that it was now in God's hands.

Later, I was told that the pressure inside the skull was no longer increasing. It was coming down. There were no new medical interventions made to explain this occurrence. The intracranial pressure became normal. The patient awoke from the coma, and recovered quickly. The patient was transferred to a regular floor and eventually discharged. I saw the patient for follow up afterward, and was amazed to find that the patient had recovered completely with no residual neurological deficits. With tears in the eyes, the parent told me that a miracle happened after we prayed in the ICU. There was complete restoration, not only of the sick and dying child, but for the entire family through the power of prayer and faith. In this particular situation, the medical institution was unable to save this patient. Everyone thought the child would die. But with divine intervention, the patient was completely cured. When I was praying for the child, another neurologist and some nurses in the room thought I was insane for praying and providing hope to this family. After the full recovery of this girl, this neurologist stated "I guess your God does have the power to heal".

Now let us apply the principles of the **RESTORATION** model to ASD, ADHD, Tourette's syndrome, OCD and other neurological/neuropsychiatric conditions. To do this, we will use the acronym **RESTORATION**. This acronym will outline specific factors that explain how children with the above conditions can be restored to health, simply, effectively and safely. Keep in mind that the recommendations below are to be thought of as one package or unit. It can only be fully effective if implemented in its entirety.

R- REST

Obtain proper sleep, at least 8 hours daily. The amount may vary between individuals, but this is the usual amount. It is important to get quality sleep *before* midnight. Sleep provides mental as well as physical restoration and healing from the daily wear and tear of life. Special hormones are released for that purpose. The body simply cannot function optimally without adequate rest. Sleep depravation can worsen anxiety, stress, headaches and seizures. Cognition and behavior will also be affected by improper sleep.

Now what can be done to help with sleep?

-Nourish your child properly (see section on nutrition). There are many food substances that directly interfere with sleep or promote problems such as gastroesophageal reflux that can interfere with sleep.

-Engage in aerobic exercise daily (walking is excellent). Video games do not count as exercise. Proper exercise can relieve stress which is very important in autism. It can allow the gut to work better (for those where constipation is a problem). Exercise can also promote better sleep.

-Make the bedroom an enticing place to sleep with as little distractions as possible. Television, videos, and Nintendo/PlayStation need to be removed from the bedroom. Avoid excessive noise, which has been shown to alter the quality of sleep. Have a comfortable mattress.

-Depending on the age of the child, identify any medical problem that may be present. You will need the help of your primary care physician. Conditions such as gastroesophageal reflux should be suspected in a young child who wakes up screaming and is irritable with daytime spitting up. Headaches, stomachaches or other pain syndromes may interfere with sleep. Seizures may disturb or prevent sleep. Children with seizures, who have warning signs known as auras especially if they occur nocturnally, may sometimes be afraid to go to sleep. Depression and other mood disorders may impair sleep.

-Consider using melatonin. This is safe, effective and natural. There is anecdotal evidence that it can help with behavior and seizures. This is over-the-counter and comes in pill or liquid form.

E-EXERCISE

Exercise is important in every aspect of health maintenance and restoration. Exercise can help our bodies physically, emotionally and mentally. Metabolism is improved, immune function is enhanced and gastrointestinal performance boosted. Exercise relieves stress. All of the above are important for autism. As mentioned, exercise does not necessarily mean running a marathon. It can entail a simple daily activity like walking. Walking is particularly helpful in that it is easy, stress-free, inexpensive, and can allow an individual to get plenty of fresh air, sunlight and improve respiratory function. Thirst sensation can increase which can lead to more water intake. Older kids and teenagers with autism often spend hours on the computer or Nintendo at the expense of good exercise. Going for a good late afternoon or early morning family walk can be good for the entire family.

## S-SUNSHINE

Sunlight is beneficial not only to plants but to humans. Many studies have documented the immune benefits of sunlight. Vitamin D production is enhanced. Mood may improve. Many children with autism, for a variety of reasons may not get the quantity of sunlight required. Because of behavioral concerns, many children with autism do not go out often. By encouraging more outdoor activities, perhaps with exercise, this requirement for optimal health can be met.

## T- TEMPERANCE

Moderation in everything is important. Temperance, in addition to moderation, conveys the idea of self-control. Self-control is important in appetite, behavior, sleep and all areas. When it comes to eating, many children with autism are said to be very picky eaters but many manage to overindulge in junk food with empty calories. This is harmful to their health. It is easier for a child with autism to become temperate if the entire family makes that a priority.

## O- OPEN-MINDEDNESS

Everyone needs to be open-minded, including the child with autism, the parents, family members, schoolteachers, therapists and clinicians. Being open-minded can provide an open door to a path that can lead to healing and restoration. Being close-minded is the surest way to fail in being made whole. Children with autism have a tendency to stick to routines and structure and engage in self-stimulatory behaviors. Partly because they feel secure with what they already know. They are scared to venture into new territories, try new foods or new activities. Parents must be the first to venture out and consider new treatment options for the sake of their children, before the children can show openness to new things.

R- RENEWAL

Everything must be renewed, body, mind, outlook and spiritual commitment. This is a prerequisite for total restoration.

A-AIR

Air is vital. It contains oxygen which is very important. Oxygen is the most abundant and vital nutrient in nature. Without it, we cannot survive for more than a few minutes. Proper air intake can be automatic if an aerobic exercise is instituted daily. Hypoxemia can impair cognition. The air that is breathed in an out of the house should be pure. Smoking is an absolute no-no around children, with or without autism. If you are a parent of a child, and you smoke, quit that habit for your child's sake, and yours. Impure air or aerial pollution is a big problem in the autism community, in that children with autism seem to have an impaired ability to get rid of any type of toxins including environmental ones. As much as possible, children with autism should be exposed to a clean environment.

## T- TRUST IN GOD

God is the ultimately healer. Only He is all powerful. Your child's doctor may be smart, well-trained, and very knowledgeable, but he does not have all the answers. Your therapist may be dedicated and empathetic but cannot heal your child. Appropriate support and therapies are useful, but God is the ultimate healer. Putting your trust in Him is a pivotal part of the **RESTORATION** model. When a child's situation seems hopeless, God is still able to restore the child to full health, *if* it is His will.

## I- INSIGHT

Always try to gain insight into your child's illness. This may take patience and planning. Every problem and every tantrum has a trigger. Even behavioral outbursts that seem to occur "out of the blue" have a trigger. In some instances, some abnormal behaviors may be attempts to communicate. Some times they are a reflection of a painful event, fear or anxiety. If as a parent you lack insight, you can ask God and He will give it to you.

## O- OPTIMISM

You should never give up. You should be hopeful and optimistic. By being optimistic you open the door of success. You can more easily be open-minded if you are optimistic. Your optimism can be contagious to your child. Optimism will drive you forward.

N- NUTRITION

Nutrition plays a vital role in autism. Very simply, we advocate making sure that all of the essential nutrients are taken including:

- Vitamins
- Minerals/trace elements
- Amino Acids
- Essential Fatty acids
- Phytochemicals
- Phytosterols
- Antioxidants
- Glyconutrients

We also recommend proper water intake. Individuals should drink approximately 6-8 glasses of water or, more precisely, the equivalent in ounces of one half the individual's weight in pounds. For instance, if the individual weighs 64 pounds, he should drink a 32 ounce bottle of water each day (that does not include other beverages). Carrying a water bottle and ensuring that it is empty before the day is over is good way to guarantee proper water intake. Avoid all toxins as much as possible. Avoid foods that are overly processed or not well tolerated:

- Dairy
- Red meats/ other processed meats
- Caffeine
- Food colors and additives

- ❑ Refined sugar
- ❑ Wheat (for some)

Eat more raw, fresh, organic and unprocessed foods. Proper nutrition should be complete and wholesome to allow the body to heal itself. We do not believe that it is necessary to over do it. Just provide the body with what it actually needs and it will do the rest. You must have faith that the body when it is given the right tools through proper nourishment, can take care of itself. It does not need us to micromanage it.

# TABLE 5
## Prescription for autism:
## RESTORATION

**Rx:** RESTORATION (TOTAL)

**Sig:**

| | |
|---|---|
| R- Rest | A-Air (fresh) |
| E- Exercise | T- Trust (in God) |
| S- Sunshine | I- Insight |
| T- Temperance | O- Optimism |
| O- Open-mindedness | N- Nutrition and Hydration |
| R- Renewal | |

**Side effects:** NONE

**Mechanism of action:** Stimulating doctors from within using biopsychosociospiritual

## BRIDGING THE GAP BETWEEN TRADITIONAL AND NON TRADITIONAL APPROACHES TO AUTISM!

PARENTS AND PHYSICIANS SHOULD WORK TOGETHER TO HELP SOLVE THE AUTISM CRISIS. Physicians should be better listeners when it comes to autism. They should be more aware of the role of nutritional therapies in autism and other disorders in general. They should be more open-minded to theories and ideas that were not taught in medical school, if they are plausible. Parents should not look down on physicians simply because they are not as well informed about particular treatment options. It is true that many physicians are close-minded when it comes to autism treatments of which they have never heard. New ideas that go against what physicians have been taught are very hard for doctors to accept or even consider, especially if they are not backed up by well designed, double-blind, placebo control studies.

When it comes to obtaining help from your doctor for your child with autism, keep the following in mind:

Be assertive but not aggressive. Do not be defensive or antagonistic
Be persistent but not overly demanding
Propose but do not impose.
Ask questions.
If you would like your physician to consider a particular treatment approach, see if you can find studies to support the effectiveness

of that treatment, and give a copy to your physician.

It is always okay to ask to be referred to a specialist or ask for a second opinion if you do not feel that your physician is getting to the bottom of things.

It is always better to work with a physician that may not be as knowledgeable about autism but is open-minded and willing to help than one that says he/she knows a lot but is close-minded to treatment options.

Be cognizant that controversies exist. When medical controversies cannot be resolved easily, it may mean that there is some truths on both sides of the fence. There may be political issues involved and confusing data that makes the topic subject to multiple explanations. You must do what you feel is best for your child bearing in mind safety issues. Traditional medicine, unfortunately, is not always as open as it should be to nutritional interventions. As far as non-conventional therapies, however, the door is left open so wide that there is room for a lot of charlatans, greedy opportunists and pseudo-scientists to creep in, preying on helpless patients and their parents. Parents should therefore always be on the alert.

Before starting a particular treatment/therapy, ask the following questions:

1- How long will the treatment/therapy last?
2- What is the expected/anticipated outcome? (try to get a range, e.g. best versus worst case scenario and in between)
3- What are the possible side effects?

4- How long should a particular treatment be continued, before deciding that it is not helpful for the child?

5- Why was that particular treatment chosen for your particular child?

**The ideal treatment is one that is effective, safe, affordable, reasonable and doable.**

<u>**SUMMARY:**</u>

The big picture for parents and physicians in treating autism should be as follows:

> - Identify etiological/causative factors as much as possible.
> - Always have a high index of suspicion for both seizures and sensory processing disorders.
> - Strengthen the immune system and make sure the gut is working well.
> - Eat properly, avoid all toxic food substances and take proper nutritional supplementation.
> - Realize that there are both primary and secondary problems in ASD. While the secondary problems must be recognized and treated, one has to specifically look for and address the primary defect for the best outcome.
> - Allow each therapeutic intervention enough time to work. In some cases this may take weeks or months. Be patient.
> - Address psychosocial factors
> - Place your ultimate trust in God, the ultimate healer.

<u>**APPENDICES**</u>

## A- FIRST AID FOR AUTISM: SURVIVAL TIPS FOR DESPERATE PARENTS

1) Try never to panic. Stay calm.
2) Find the underlying cause(s) specifically and as soon as possible (see example below):
3) Start treatment as soon as possible.
4) Explore every option, but one at a time, with the most likely option first.
5) Give each treatment ample time to work (in some case several months) but know when to "call it quits" on a particular treatment option.
6) Never ever give up and be optimistic always.
7) Be a good observer. Take into account every effect of treatment whether beneficial or adverse
8) Acknowledge the fact that a treatment that works for one child may not necessarily apply to your child, or may even cause adverse effects. Focus on your child.
9) Be persistent with treatment.
10) Take into account the body's God-given ability to heal itself and the brain's natural course of maturation.
11) Seek appropriate help.

The following example pertains to an exacerbation or persistence of self-stimulatory behavior:

- ❑ Always keep a log or calendar of self stimulatory behaviors, anything that the child ate or drank, any infections/fever that precipitated the events, any particular drug or natural supplements. Although natural supplements are safe, some may not always be the right for a given child. Also make notes of any environmental changes, as well as psychosocial stressors.

- ❑ Remove any perceived stresses or triggers from the child's environment.

- ❑ It is important for the parents themselves not to be stressed since the child can feel on the parents' stress, which could aggravate the self-stimulatory behaviors. At times it may mean completely ignoring the self-stimulatory behaviors. Unlike some forms of epileptic motor seizures that can be harmful if they persist more than several minutes, this is not the case with self stimulatory behaviors. They may be annoying, they may appear bizarre, you may want to remove them, but the fact is that they do not harm the brain. That means there is time to patiently work at removing the stressors.

- ❑ It is of vital importance to make sure that the child's diet is healthy, well-balanced and well supplemented with the appropriate nutritional supplements. In many instances, that alone can completely eliminate the self-stimulatory behaviors. Metabolic issues, detoxification problems, and various infections (bacterial and fungal/yeast) can trigger tics and should be appropriately identified and treated.

❑ Know your child's mode of sensory learning and be aware of any sensory processing difficulties that are present. For instance if your child has a sound sensitivity or, what is commonly referred to as painful hearing, it is possible in that an exacerbation of self-stimulatory behaviors may be the result of over exposure to certain harmful sounds. The same can apply for visual sensory disturbances.

Since some self-stimulatory behaviors may be self-soothing mechanisms, it only makes sense that before you try to extinguish a particular behavior, you find a replacement behavior that is also soothing.

## B- GENETIC AND CHROMOSOMAL PROBLEMS NOTED IN AUTISM:

Del 1q43, del 15q, interstitial del 17 (p11.2), t(1;7;21), 3p-, 5p+, 8p-, 17p-, 18q-,

t(5;6)(q13;p23),t(3;12)(p26.3;q23.3),t(X;8)(p22.13; q22.1), t(22,13), t(1;15)(p35;q1233),

Tri 21, tri 22, partial tri 16p,

Iso Y dup q11-21, inv Y(p11;q11), iso Y dup q11-21,

Monosomy (5 pter-5p15.3),

XXX, XXY, XYY, XXYY, Large Y,

Adrenomyloneuropathy, Angelman's syndrome, Basal cell nevus syndrome, Ceroid storage disease, Cohen syndrome, Cornelia de Lange Syndrome, Duchene's muscular dystrophy, Fragile X syndrome, Goldenhar's syndrome, Histidinemia, Hurler's syndrome, Hypomelanosis of Ito, Joubert's syndrome, Mobius syndrome, Neurofibromatosis, Neurolipodisis, Noonan's syndrome, Oculocutaneous albinism, Peter's Plus syndrome, Phenylketonuria (untreated), Sanfilippo's syndrome, type A, Shprintzen's syndrome, Marshall-Smith syndrome, Tuberous Sclerosis, Williams syndrome and XLMR with Marfanoid habitus. (Textbook of Pediatric Neuropsychiatry).

# C- GLOSSARY OF IMPORTANT TERMINOLOGY

**ABA** (Applied Behavioral Analysis): A form of behavioral modification therapy, usually intensive, where behavior is taught by discrete trials. Lovaas is the most popular form.

**Asperger's Syndrome**: A higher functioning form of autism where an individual typically has normal to above intelligence. They may have focused precocious levels of interest and clumsiness. There are significant social deficits present.

**Casein**: A protein found in dairy. Some children with autism improve when this is removed from the diet. Intestinal symptoms and recurrent infections, as well as behavioral changes are common with casein sensitivity.

**Chelation**: A process where an agent is given orally, intravenously or trandermally to remove toxic heavy metals (e.g. mercury) stored in the body. Examples of chelating agents commonly used in autism include DMSA and DMPS.

**Gluten**: A protein found in wheat, oat and barley. Some children with autism improve when this is removed from the diet. Individuals with celiac disease also do not tolerate gluten. Intestinal symptoms are common with gluten sensitivity

**Gut dysbiosis**: An imbalance of gut flora that allows pathogens such as certain species of yeast to overgrow while useful organisms such as probiotics are deficient. This may result in secondary problems of behavior and neurological function.

**Iatrogenic**: Medical condition induced or caused by improper treatment. Examples include ailments caused by side effects of drugs. Some medical treatments may cause ailments that are far worse then the conditions that are being treated. This may also be the case in autism.

**Kanner's autism**: Primary or classic autism. Usually it has a more severe presentation.

**Leaky gut syndrome**: A condition of the gut whereby there is comprise of the barrier function of the gut wall causing large molecules and toxins to pass through the gut wall. Gut dysfunction results in immune disturbances, food allergies, stress on the liver and further compromise of gastrointestinal function. This may contribute to autoimmune disturbances.

**Metallothionein promotion therapy**. A popular form of "natural chelation" where zinc is given for several weeks along with vitamins to correct functioning of a protein called metallothionein involved in regulation of copper and zinc levels.

**PDD** (Pervasive Developmental Disorder): A term introduced in the 1980s to describe a class of 5 apparently related conditions: autistic disorder, Rett syndrome, Childhood Disintegrative disorder, Asperger's syndrome.

**Rett's Syndrome**: A neurodegenerative condition affecting females. They usually start with a head size that is becomes smaller, with characteristic hand ringing and progressive development of autistic symptoms. Seizures are common. Any female child with autism, with a small head should be evaluated for Rett syndrome.

**Regressive autism**: A form of autism that is acquired. It occurs in a child who initially was progressing normally. Implications for this form of autism may be very different from the type that starts congenitally (from birth).

**Specific carbohydrate diet**: A dietary approach that is based on the idea that an increased carbohydrate load is responsible for increased stress on the gastrointestinal tract. Therefore, eliminating those specific carbohydrates can allow the gut to heal. Initially developed for conditions such as Crohn's disease and ulcerative colitis, many children with autism have been placed on this diet.

**Sulfation Defect**: A dysfunction of an enzyme called phenosulfotransferase which causes abnormalities in detoxification.

**Sulfonation-** replenishing sulfur to allow detoxification to occur.

**REFERENCES:**

## ALTERNATIVE THERAPIES

<u>Commonly used herbal medicines in the United States: a review.</u>  S. Bent, MD ad R. Ko, PharmD, PhD.  American Journal of Medicine.  Volume 116, Number 7, April 1, 2004.
<u>Herbal Cures for Common Ailments.</u>  Jim O'Brien.  Globe Digests.  1997.
<u>The Antioxidant Miracle</u>. Lester Packer, PhD & Carol Colman.  1999.
<u>Treatment choice is ultimately the patient's.</u>  M. Fleming, MD.  American Medical News.  Page 19, October 4, 2004.

## GLUTEN/CASEIN-FREE DIET

Adv. Biochem. Psychopharmacol. 28: 27-643.
Autism 1999; 3:45-65.
Brain Dysfunction, 3 (1990): 308-19.
Brain Research 412 (1987) p. 68-72.
Dev Brain Dysfunct 7 (1994) p. 71-85.
Journal of Applied Nutrition 42 no. 1 (1990) 1-11.
Oski, Frank A. (1992) Don't Drink Your Milk! New Frightening Medical Facts About
the Worlds Most Overrated Nutrient, 9th Edition. Teach Services: Burshton, NY.
Panksepp J Trends in Neurosciences 2 (1979) p. 174-177.

## AUTISM EPIDEMIC

Blaxil MF- Public Health Rep-01-NOV-2004; 119 (6): 536-51.

CDC, April 2000. "Prevalence of Autism in Brick Township, New Jersey, 1998: Community Report".
Croen LA- J Autism and Developmental Disorders 01- June-2002; 32 (3):217-24.
Disabilities Education Act, Table, AA11. pp 6-21.
Fombonne E- J Autism Dev Disord-01-AUG-2003; 33(4):365-82.
Lancet 1997; 350:1761-6.
Merrick J- Int J Adolesc Med Health – 01 – Jan – 2004; 16 (1):75-8.
22nd Annual Report to Congress on the Implementation of the individuals with Pediatrics Vol. 107 No. 2 February 2001, pp. 411-412.
U.S. News & World Report, June 19, 2000 p.47.
Yeargin-Allsopp M-JAMA – 1 – Jan-2003; 289 (1): 49-55.

## B6 AND MAGNESIUM

Ann NY Acad Sci 1990; 585: 250-60.
Biol Psychiatry 1991 May 1; 29 (9) 931-41.
Dev Med Child Neurol 1989 Dec; 31 (6): 721-7.
J. Autism Dev Disord 1995 Oct; 25 (5): 481-93.
J. Autism Dev Disord 1998 Dec; 28 (6) 581-2.
J. Child Neurol 1988; 3 Suppl: S68-72.

## AUTISM AND SEIZURES

Advances in Neurology 1986; 501-12.
Arch Neurol 1988;45:666-668.
Epilepsia, 1989, 30, 90-93 (improvement of seizures with DMG).
J AM Acad Child Psychiatry 1990:29z;127-129.
New England Journal of Medicine 1982, 307, 1081-1082 (improvement of seizures with DMG).

Pediatrics 1999 Sep; 104 # 405-18 (82% of children with ASD have clinically relavent abnormality on EEG (MEG).

## **GUT PROBLEMS (DYSBIOSIS) IN AUTISM**

Acta Paediatr 1998 Aug; 87 (8) 836-4.
Clin Sci (Colch) 2000 Aug; 99 (2): 93-1-4.
Dig Dis Sci. 2000 Apr;45(4)723-9.
Gut 2002 May; 50 Suppl 3: III60-III54.
J. Assoc Acad Minor Phys. 1998; 9 (1):9-15.
J. Child Neurol. 2000 Jul: 15(7):429-35.
J. Pediatr 1999 Nove;135 (5):559-63.
Lancet. 1998 Feb 28; 351 (9103): 637-41.
Lancet. 2000 Aug 26; 356 (9231).
Mol Psychiatry 2000;7 (4):375-82.
Pediatr. 2001 Mar; 138(3): 366-72.
Proc Natl Acad Sci USA 1999 Oct 12;96 (21) 12012-7.
Toxicol Ind Health 1998 Jul-Aug; 14 (4) 553-63.

## **DETOXIFICATION PROBLEMS**

J. Nutri Enviro Med 2000; 10 (1):25-32.
J. Orthomolec. Med., 8(4) 198-200.
Toxicology 1996; 111:43-65.

## **FOOD SENSITIVITIES/ADDITIVES**

Annals of Allergy 1994, 72(5) 462-468.
Annals of Allergy 1994, 73 (3) 215-19.
J. Orthomolec 1993. Med., 8 (4).
Panminerva Med 1995 Sep; 37(3): 137-41.
Scand J Educaional Res 1995; 39: 223-36.

## THIMEROSAL AND AUTISM

Molecular Psychiatry 2004, 1-13. Neurotoxic effects of postnatal Thimerosal are mouse strain dependent.

## AUTOIMMUNITY AND AUTISM

Pediatrics 01-NOV-2003; 112 (5): E420 Increased prevalence of familial autoimmunity with pervasive developmental disorders.

## BOOKS:

1) A Guide to Scientific Nutrition For Autism and Related Conditions. By Kirkman Laboratories.

2) Behavioral Intervention for Young Children with Autism. By Catherine Maurice.

3) Beyond the Wall. Personal Experiences with Autism and Asperger Syndrome. By Stephen Shore.

4) Biological Treatments for Autism and PDD. By William Shaw, Ph.D.

5) Children with Starving Brains: A Medical Treatment Guide for Autism Spectrum Disorder. By Jacquelyn McCandless, MD.

6) Facing Autism: Giving Parents Reasons for Hope and Guidance for Help. By Lyn M. Hamilton.

7) Oski, Frank A. (1992) Don't Drink Your Milk! New Frightening Medical Facts About the Worlds Most Overrated Nutrient, 9<sup>th</sup> Edition. Teach Services: Burshton, NY.

8) Special Diets for Special Kids. By Lisa Lewis, Ph.D.

9) The Textbook of Pediatric Neuropsychiatry. By Edward Coffey, MD & Roger A. Brumback, MD. American Psychiatric Press, Inc. 1998.

10) Thinking in Pictures: And Other Reports From My Life with Autism. By Temple Grandin.

11) Unraveling the Mystery of Autism and Pervasive Developmental Disorder: A Mother's Story of Research and Recovery. By Karyn Seroussi.

12) What Your Doctor May Not Tell you About Children's Vaccinations. By Stephanie Cave, M.D., F.A.A.F.P.

**<u>WEBSITES:</u>**

www.autism-alabama.org
www.autism.com/ari
www.vaporia.com/autism/
www.gnd.org
www.gfcfdiet.org
www.AutismNDI.com

# ABOUT THE AUTHOR:

Dr. Jean-Ronel Corbier is a board certified Pediatric Neurologist who specializes in the treatment of autism. His background is unique in that he grew up in several different countries. He lived in Africa with his parents as missionaries for 7 years. This exposure greatly broadened his perspective on life. He went to medical school at Michigan State University College of Human Medicine. He completed his neurology training at the University of Cincinnati and Children's Hospital of Cincinnati. He has also completed neurology electives at Johns Hopkins, the Mayo Clinic and the University of Michigan. While in medical school, he enrolled concurrently in a graduate program in Health and Humanities. This gave him the opportunity to work on several projects with alternative health professionals. Dr. Jean-Ronel Corbier has been investigating the role of nutrition in the treatment of various neurological disorders and might be thought of as a pediatric nutritional neurologist. This background along with Dr. Corbier's strong Christian faith, gives him a broad and unique perspective on the complex disorder of autism. Dr. Jean-Ronel Corbier currently practices pediatric neurology in Montgomery, Alabama. His wife is a Pediatrician, and they have one son.

Dr. Corbier can be reached at (334) 396-0761.

# Other Pertinent Information About the Author

## Personal

Birthday:        September 10, 1966
Birthplace:      New York City, New York

## Education

1997-2000       Fellowship, Children's Hospital Medical Center
                Pediatric Neurology
1997-1998       Fellowship, University of Cincinnati
                Adult Neurology
1995-1997       Residency, Hurley Medical Center
                Pediatrics
                Flint, Michigan
Jan. 1995       Elective/Neurology
                Mayo Clinic
                Rochester, Minnesota
Dec. 1994       Elective/ Neurology
                John's Hopkins University
June 1992       Elective/Neurology
                University of Michigan
1990-1995       MD, Michigan State University-- College of Human Medicine
                East Lansing, Michigan
1990-1995       Graduate Studies, Michigan State Universty
                East Lansing, Michigan
Summer 1991     Medical Ethics & History of Healthcare
                University of London
1985-1989       BA, Andrews University
                Biology
                Berrien Springs, Michigan

# **Employment**

| | |
|---|---|
| Nov. 02-present | Pediatric Neurology, Private Practice |
| | Montgomery, Alabama |
| Mar. 02-present | Children's Rehabilitative Services/Neurology Clinic |
| | Montgomery, Alabama |
| Oct. 02-Nov. 02 | Pediatric Neurology, Pediatric Specialists of Montgomery |
| | Montgomery, Alabama |
| 1998-2000 | Director, Neuroscience/Pediatric Neurology Clerkship |
| | Cincinnati, Ohio |
| 1993 | Teaching Assistant |
| | Berrien Springs, Michigan |
| 1987-1989 | Nursing Assistant |
| | Berrien Springs, Michigan |
| 1986-1989 | Curator/Biological Museum-- Andrews University |
| | Berrien Springs, Michigan |
| 1987 | Literature Evangelist/SDA Church |
| | Washington, DC |

# **Honors**

| | |
|---|---|
| 2002 | Board Certification |
| | Neurology with Special Qualification in Child Neurology |
| 1998 | Adult Neurology 'Rock" Award |
| 1994 | AOA Nomination |
| 1994 | Seventh-Day Adventist General Conference Scholarship |
| 1990-1994 | EOP Fellowship |
| 1993 | Interdisciplinary Health & Humanities Scholarship |
| 1993 | Scholarship for Dual Degree Medical Students |
| 1991 | Phi Beta Delta Honor Society for International Scholar |
| 1989 | Tri Beta Biological Honor Society |

# Extracurricular & Community Activities

| | |
|---|---|
| 2000 | Director, Health & Temperance Department |
| | First Church |
| | Cincinnati, Ohio |
| 1999 | Elder, North Star Seventh-Day Adventist Church (SDA) |
| | Covington, Kentucky |
| 1995 | Director, Religious Liberty Department |
| | Fairhaven SDA Church |
| | Flint, Michigan |
| 1993-1994 | Volunteer, Lansing Health Screening Program |
| | Lansing, Michigan |
| 1992-1994 | Member, Center for Meaning & Health |
| | East Lansing, Michigan |
| 1988-1989 | Public Relations Director, Pre-Med Minority Club |
| | Andrews University |
| | Berrien Springs, Michigan |
| 1978-1985 | Missionary/Leper Colony |
| | Central and West Africa |

# Memberships

Child Neurology Society
American Academy of Neurology
Neurology Society of Alabama
Medical Association of the State of Alabama
Member, American Board of Medical Specialists

To order additional copies of:

# Solving the Enigma of Autism

Call 334-418-0088
Or please visit our website at
www.UfomaduConsulting.com